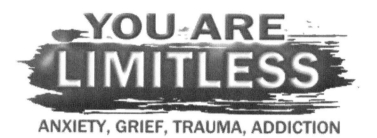

# YOU ARE LIMITLESS

## ANXIETY, GRIEF, TRAUMA, ADDICTION

### 7 INSPIRING STORIES OF HOPE & HEALING

KATE CHAMPION

**You Are Limitless**
Anxiety, Grief, Trauma, Addiction
7 Inspiring Stories of Hope & Healing

Published by Mountain Morning Press, Ltd.
ISBN: 978-1-7344806-6-5 (paperback)
ISBN: 978-1-7344806-7-2 (ePub)
Also available for Kindle

Design & pre-press: Lighthouse24

*To Mother Nature,
and all those in pursuit of healing...*

# CONTENTS

# INTRODUCTION

*"At the core of your being you are spiritual, limitless, and beautiful..."*
— Debasish Mridha

AHH, THIS BOOK... be it a trip to the beach, the first few steps on a trail head, or the beginning of a new chapter—we just don't know where our adventures will take us. This truth has been pertinent, particularly in my case. We can have the best ideas, hopes, plans, dreams, and intentions. Yet, like the seasons, time and life evolves. Sometimes moving along as intended. Sometimes throwing us a curve ball or two...

Welcome to the second book in the *Never Too Late* series. I continue to be honored and inspired by so many accounts of real, everyday people doing incredible things. This book continues in the same spirit. Within the following pages you will find a compilation of inspirational stories narrated by some amazing real-life people. No glitz, glamor, fake, or fabricated anything.

It takes incredible courage to share in such an open and vulnerable way. As part of the interview/ publication process the option for anonymity was offered; accordingly, some people have asked to remain nameless. Their wishes have been respected and pseudonyms have been created.

This might be a good moment for a disclaimer or a reader alert. There is some tough stuff in the pages ahead. We take a deep dive into topics such as grief, anxiety, addiction, trauma, and discrimination. We touch upon lifestyle concerns such as obesity, stress, and autoimmune disorders. Remember, these are real accounts, raw and honest.

Woven within every story you will also discover seeds of wisdom, compassion, encouragement, hope, and support. You will learn about how nature together with movement (walking, hiking, climbing, etc.) has, and continues to be, an integral part of their healing process.

For *Never Too Late* that glimmer of inspiration came from a beginner backpacking trip I gifted myself for my 55th birthday. Through that serendipitous experience, I connected with and built a community with other later-in-life athletes— runners, hikers, swimmers, mountain climbers— people who continue to thrive in their 60s, 70s, and 80s. Consequently, my desire to thrive and my passion for everything outdoorsy has exploded.

While all the accounts in *Never Too Late* are truly inspirational, the story of one woman—Anne 'Annie' Crispin Taylor—took my sense of admiration to a whole new level. As a psychotherapist who works primarily with grief, loss, trauma, anxiety, and addiction, I have the honor of coming alongside much human suffering—heartbreak, loss, horrors of every shape and size—that people, through no fault of their own, have endured and survived.

Something about Annie's journey deeply resonated with me... I'm sure you know: it's the way we feel when our hearts shift a little and a part of us stops to pause for a moment—allowing time and space to open— to truly hear and see another human being in all their glory. For those who haven't read *Never Too Late*, here's a bit about Annie's story (adapted from *Never Too Late: Inspiration, Motivation, and Sage Advice from 7 Later-In-Life Athletes* by Kate Champion, 2020).

*Annie grew up in California. Not particularly a 'sporty' child in the traditional sense. Horses were her passion throughout high school. With the transition to college and adulting, Annie left horses behind and took the opportunity to travel in Europe for a year, returning to the States in her early 20s. Annie married in her 30s, becoming the caregiver for three children. When her youngest child was eight, Annie went back to school for her bachelor's degree.*

*Annie found running in college. She recalls, "It helped to take my mind off all the studies. I'd take a break and go run." Annie lived near the mountains. Naturally, trail running became a big part of her life, and she spent many hours running on the trails with her dog. Annie found trail running so freeing, "I*

*would go out there, and not think about anything."*
*When Annie turned 50, she decided to run her first*
*100-mile race. She enjoyed the experience—and the*
*challenge so much—she committed to running one*
*100-mile race every year for the decade.*

*In January the following year, after struggling to*
*figure out some physical health symptoms, Annie*
*was diagnosed with squamous cell carcinoma, an*
*aggressive cancer of the mouth. That February, she*
*had surgery to remove the tumor. During the process*
*all the lymph nodes in her throat and neck were*
*removed. March saw the beginning of six weeks of*
*grueling radiation treatment. Annie recalls, "The*
*treatments were draining and my energy was*
*extremely low."*

*Annie's recovery process included learning how*
*to eat again, trying to recover all the weight she had*
*lost, and physical therapy to help improve the*
*mobility of her arms, head, and neck. Although the*
*surgery had left Annie with some limitations, she*
*continued to be diligent about her daily exercises.*

*Remarkably, none of this slowed Annie down.*
*The year following her surgery, fueled by a diet of*
*baby food, Annie continued to train for—and*
*complete—her second 100-mile race. In 2016, Annie*
*ran three 100-mile races. And then, three more 100-*
*milers in 2017, which fulfilled her dream: to finish*
*her tenth 100-mile race before her 60th birthday.*
*Annie described the "huge joy!" she felt that day,*

*sharing that, "Overcoming cancer has been one of the hardest things I have ever done."*

Annie continued, *"I get so much joy out of running. I live near a beautiful park which has access to eight miles of trail. I can lace up, head out the door, run half a mile down the street and I'm in the park. I feel a strong emotional connection to this park. To nature. I can see Mount Hood off in the distance, great views of the city, and all the bridges that span the river. Day or night, it's so beautiful! Having a beautiful place to run inspires me…"*

And there it is—bam! In the rich soil of inspiration, mixed with compassion and awe, the seed for this book was planted. Annie's story. Her passion, perseverance, recovery, and connection with the natural world captured my curiosity and became the essence of this work.

As I curate a bit of Annie's story for you, I remember feeling humbled, inspired, honored, and incredibly grateful to be a witness to, and share, Annie's story. I hope that the strength, courage, and tenacity of this remarkable woman, along with the phenomenal stories from the real-life warriors spotlighted in *You Are Limitless* will touch and inspire you. Within these pages, I hope you will learn how to connect with your limitless nature, empower yourself through the use of movement, and be inspired to explore the healing power of the natural world.

## The Project

If you have read any of my other work, you will know that I love to mix inspirational stories about real people with practical tips, tools, and resources as well as actionable strategies you can learn and practice. This book continues in that tradition, with chapters dedicated to spotlighting seven incredible people with powerful accounts of adversity, despair, healing, and recovery—woven in with messages about mindset, determination, and why nature and movement are vital components of the healing and recovery process.

I'll start with a bit about how this project has enriched my healing journey, and then introduce the incredible people who have been so generous with their time, energy, and deeply personal stories.

Some things are difficult to put into words, like the way colors shift in the pre-dawn sky, or the feeling of being in the midst of a stand of majestic old growth pines, or the way layers of grief or fear or anger can dissipate like the morning mist as I move through the woods. Equally challenging is the expression of felt senses like joy, awe, wonder, and deep loss—all sensations that fill the mind, body, and heart.

Recently, during some work with my therapist, I uncovered a very early memory. A little girl—probably around two—standing out in the spring sunshine feeding the lambs. You see, when I was young my parents owned and operated a small farm with chickens, lambs, and goats. This memory brought feelings of warmth, safety, comfort, and peace. Yet, behind me in the house, things were not so easy, bright, or fun: there was a darkness. It was during this time that my father died. As if that weren't enough, his death threw our family—my mother—into a tailspin of chaos, anguish, and frankly, hardship for many years. That memory of the little girl with the lambs felt like an "aha moment." My therapist commented, "Maybe that's why your connection with nature is so strong, so important, so vital?" Indeed, throughout what I call my "challenging first quarter" (the first 25 years of my life), I sought solace and found great comfort in nature, as I still do to this day.

Not surprising when you think about it. By design we are intricately connected with the natural world. We depend on oxygen, sunlight, and nutrients which come from the soil. Moreover, physically, we are mostly water mixed with other living matter (microbes, organisms, bacteria, etc.). We have cycles and systems which are strongly linked to the seasons, daylight, and temperature. The topics of nature and natural science are vast, way beyond my expertise and the scope of this book. However, in the Resources section you will find some of the books and podcasts that have been helpful in my journey.

Compared to *Never Too Late* the conversations in this book have come along quite organically by way of Facebook, podcasts, and word of mouth. From my adventuring, hiking, and outdoor pursuits, I have built a community of likeminded people. I know where to go and what to listen for. I have an ear for—and a love of—connecting with real people and their inspiring stories. As a more established author this time, I am not grappling around in the dark quite so much as when I was just starting out.

For this current book I continue with the question-and-answer format, with the exception of the final story: my conversation with Dr. Betty Holston Smith, an 81-year-old woman who is an absolute inspiration. More on Dr. Betty later.

Heading through the chapters in logical order, the first conversation comes from me, Kate Champion. As you will learn in my chapter, I too have a story; however, I had not considered sharing it. Yet here we are... It seems that the world conspired, serving me an opportunity for which I am grateful. My intention? To inspire, support, and offer a glimmer of hope.

Next you will meet Lisa Smith, whose journey started in childhood with an intense battle with addiction—specifically alcohol. Lisa was incredibly open about her experiences. No sugar coating it here... Lisa takes us from the depths of addiction— and her perception of waking up in jail with blood on her hands—to reclaiming her life and the joy of sobriety with the help of a very long walk in nature.

Then the spotlight moves to Dierdre Wolownick, a remarkable woman who tells an unusual story about a different kind of survival. I came across Dierdre while reading a magazine article about "later-in-life" athletes. Her passion is rock climbing, and at 71 years old, Dierdre is the oldest woman to scale the 3000-foot rockface of El Capitan in Yosemite National Park. Dierdre is also a writer. As a prelude to our conversation, I picked up her memoir *The Sharp End of Life: A Mother's Story* and read it from cover to cover. Her resilience and deep connection with the natural world glistened through the pages. "Ahh…" I thought, "she would be perfect…" I found her profile on Instagram and crafted a message; soon we had connected and scheduled a time to talk.

Next you will hear from frontline healthcare provider Sally Adams. I remember initially connecting with Sally, who was concerned that her story "wasn't enough"—bad enough, tough enough, tragic enough… After a couple of minutes, it was clear that Sally and her story were absolutely perfect. Why? Because her experiences, particularly over the past couple of years working on the frontlines, as a nurse in an emergency department during the height of the COVID pandemic, are unprecedented. The effects—emotional, physical, psychological—this had on her, and many other healthcare workers' lives, are huge and merit communication. Additionally, Sally's story highlights the many twists and turns debilitating anxiety can take, and how she used movement and nature to bring her back from the edge.

At this point, you may be thinking, "Hey, what about men? Where are their stories?" That is a great question. For this book, the focus on females was not intentional. However, as a therapist, I know that generally, women are more likely to share their experiences and seek help. Truthfully, men were not rushing to respond to my call for project participants. I needed a man... (I am happily married—no pun intended!) Enter Will Sprouse, who had been out there in my peripheral vision and was featured in a couple of articles I had read. Coincidently, one of the members of the *Back of the Pack* Facebook community had posted a link to an "amazing story"— a podcast featuring "Iron Will." Riveted, I listened to his story. Will had survived a horrendous motorbike crash, coming back from a "you'll never walk again" prognosis to running 100-mile trail races. Then, a couple of years later, he suffered a major stroke and, once again, rehabbed himself using nature as a partner in his healing process. Yes, Will was perfect. *Back of the Pack* member Scott Hagerty connected me with Will, who graciously agreed to be in the spotlight. Thanks, Scott!

Next you'll meet Janie Baxter, who responded to a post I made in a hiking group I belong to. From her email I sensed that a part of her was unsure—even scared—about making the inquiry, yet another part of her felt like it was important that she share her story. Have a voice. Help others. Janie's story starts in childhood where patterns of abuse, neglect, and violence were seeded early in life. As a young adult, she unwittingly re-experienced these blueprints. The Post-Traumatic Stress Disorder (PTSD) progressed for several decades, replaying and repeating in an abusive marriage. Today—thankfully—with the help of nature, walking, hiking, and spirituality, Janie's voice is honored as she shares her powerful message of hope, healing, and recovery.

Coming full circle in this introduction, we are back to Dr. Betty Holston Smith. Dr. Betty's name came up during the reading and research phase of this project. The search terms "nature and healing and movement" suggested her book *Lifestyle by Nature: One Woman's Break from the Unhealthy Herd to Roam Forever Healthy in Nature's Lifestyle Change Herd.* I tore through her book and begged (I have no pride…) for an interview. Her response was, "Thank you for writing to me and for your very kind words. I would love to hear more about your interesting book…" I was thrilled! Dr. Betty is an absolute inspiration. She has done it all—teaching, adventuring, writing, running. Through it all she has remained true to her beliefs around health, fitness, family, and nature. Dr. Betty, in her eighth decade, continues to run more than 80 miles a week!

Dr. Betty tells us about growing up in a family

with strong values around nature and education. She talks about segregation, desegregation, and discrimination. In her 20s, Dr. Betty battled a revolving door of obesity, diet pills, more weight gain, more fad diets, and more diet pills until she said, "No more!" From that moment, Dr. Betty has shaped her life around nature, nature's wisdom, and "going with the flow of things." In one of our exchanges, Dr. Betty shared that "Nobody has ever been interested in my whole story—just bits and pieces." She continued, stating, "Over the years, it has been frustrating." Once again, the stars aligned. I feel honored and privileged to be in the position to spotlight—and do due diligence—to Dr. Betty's amazing life. Accordingly, Dr. Betty's story comes to you in full unabridged glory.

Following Dr. Betty, you will find the "practical" chapters. There is a chapter about movement where I cover a bit about the science and why movement is so important in the healing and recovery process. Next you will find a chapter titled *Mindset: Lemons to Lemonade.* Here we look at what mindset is, why it's important, and of course I share lots of practical tips and strategies designed to shift unhelpful mindsets (our lemons if you like...) into more helpful mentalities. Finally, there's a chapter asking the question *Why Nature?* Hopefully, after reading all the inspirational stories about healing and recovery the answer to that query will be crystal clear. However, just in case, I want to ensure you have plenty of information and enough resources (books, podcasts, websites, etc.) to help you along the way...

To sum up, my mission in life is to support, inspire, and explore. Whether it's via counseling, coaching, consulting, books, groups, podcasts, or traveling, that is always my aim. I sincerely hope that through the heartfelt accounts of struggle and triumph spotlighted in the following pages you will embrace the support, allow a seed of inspiration to ignite, commit to healing, and explore your limitless nature.

## Final Business

- The order of the questions was the same for each conversation except, as mentioned, Dr. Betty.

- I love quotes. There are quotes scattered throughout the book. You will find quotes from the world at large, some of my favorite quotes, and words of wisdom taken directly from the conversations.

- You are getting 95 percent of what I got from the interviewees. If I didn't get an answer, you will know that too.

- Each conversation has gone through an editing process simply to help with flow and readability.

- Remember, some people have given permission to use their full names while others have chosen to remain anonymous. Please respect their privacy.

- In the back of the book, you will find some resources. I have included many of the resources mentioned in the chapters along with things I have personally found helpful.

- There are two free downloads. Your gift copy of *A Pocket Guide to Hiking, Running, & Backpacking: Safety Tips and Strategies for You and the Folks Back Home* by Kate Champion, plus my *How To Find a Therapist* resource.

- There is a note of thanks. Gratitude is a value of mine, and it can play an important role in the healing process.

- Lastly, stop by the *Final Words* page. Remember to follow Kate Champion Author on Facebook and Instagram. And, if you find my books helpful—which I hope you do— please spread the word: tell a friend, write a review, like and/or share. Thank you!

———

# KATE CHAMPION

Author, adventurer, therapist—shares her story of healing from grief, loss, trauma, and a debilitating autoimmune disorder— through movement and nature

> *"I believe that we have to start with ourselves, that the journey begins on the inside, and the answers come from within. Getting clear about what you want, what you need, what you're willing to do—and what you're unwilling to do—is a good starting point."*
>
> – Kate Champion

**THE WRITING LIFE** is full of twists, turns, and challenges. Getting this book out into the world was no exception. For many reasons, this was a tough one. I considered throwing in the towel on several occasions. This feeling was particularly strong when—with a final round of edits scheduled and formatters booked—a decision was made to pull a chapter.

This action left me with one of those, "Now what?" dilemmas. Of course, I had choices. Do I go with six people? Could I find someone else? Do I give up, and send my apologies to all the people who had so courageously showed up to tell their stories? Or, hmm, could I tell my personal story? While, clearly, I have a story, it was never my intention to share it. Yet here we are…

All said and done, I feel glad, proud, and honest—authentic. I'm glad that I didn't scramble to throw together a filler story. During the writing process, I connected with feelings of pride—and "okay-ness"—as I realized how much I have worked through. I think the authenticity comes from feeling bigger (as opposed to smaller), as I am finally okay with holding my head up high and saying, "Yep, this is me…"

Although I don't believe our past defines us, I do believe that our stories are woven into our physical and mental fabric through feelings, memories, beliefs, and thoughts. To be comfortable enough in my own skin to shine the spotlight in the dark corners feels freeing, like I am shedding the last traces of a burden. So, thank you! Thank you for picking up this book, reading, spending your precious time, and working so hard toward your own healing journey.

### Kate C

*Tell me a bit about you and your background.*

I was born and raised in England in a small rural village about an hour to the south of London. My father was an entrepreneur, with fingers in lots of pies. We lived on a small farm, where we raised chickens and sheep. I have a lovely photo of my mum and me outside, and we're sitting on the doorstep in the sunshine. I'm probably two and a half, toddling around exploring. There are flowers, colors, and honestly a genuine look of joy on smiling faces.

The only picture I have of my dad is also an outside scene. Still small, I am on the back of a pony—no idea where the shot was taken. Maybe we had ponies? My father, tall, slender, with dark hair was right there by my side.

My mother was a journalist. Father would work the farm and Mother would commute into London for work. I am guessing, due to farm life, we were outside a lot, playing, checking on animals, and collecting eggs.

Recently I had a memory of being a small child. A clear image of little me, at the fence, feeding the sheep and lambs. In England we have a breakfast cereal called Weetabix (palm sized wheat biscuits deliciously crunchy without milk, a soggy mess once milk is added). I would balance a couple of the crunchy bars in my small, chubby hands and offer them to the sheep. In the memory, I get the feeling it was early spring—makes sense with the lambs... Spring is still my favorite time of year.

I have a younger brother. As kids—older elementary school age, different village, different house—we had a lot of freedom. Free rein to do typical kid stuff, playing outside, riding bikes, swimming. I remember long, endless summer days when "go outside and play" was the expectation.

My mum loved flowers. Later, in my early teens, I remember her on her knees weeding and prepping the soil for spring bulbs. Tulips. Daffodils. The arrival of crocuses and bluebells was always a cause for celebration.

As a family, there was no organized outdoorsy stuff—I don't think there was time. Consequently, I learned to experience the natural world quite organically, with little snippets here and there.

I've always been a runner. First road, then—later in life—trail running. Interestingly, my connection with nature and the natural world didn't really begin to bloom until my mid-50s when I added back-packing adventures to my life. I love being outdoors. Physically, emotionally, experientially—being immersed in the woods for days has taken that connection to a whole new level.

*Diving into the tough topic, tell me a bit about your personal journey/experience.*

I often joke that the first quarter of my life was rocky, and that, now, as I head into the final quarter of my life—60 and beyond—life has hit a sweet spot. Smoothed out a bit. Yes, of course, curveballs still come my way, yet today I am better at dodging, weaving, and recovering.

Amidst the lambs and the sunshine, it seems my parents had a tumultuous relationship, agitated by money struggles, depression, and two small children.

One evening there was a particularly intense argument, so nasty that my mother left the house. The argument continued by phone—you know, big feelings, raised voices, threats.

At some point during the night my father consumed a lethal combination of alcohol and barbiturates. Overdose? Suicide? Intentional? Cry for help? No one really knows…

I was two and a half, my brother was a baby. I have the sense that there must have been a lot of shame around his death. No one talked about it. Any mention of "Dad" was shrouded in thick, awkward silence. The stories I did glean were concocted, a cover up to save face or protect or deny. When I did ask questions about how he died, lung cancer or tuberculosis were described as the cause of death, then the subject was quickly changed. I learned the truth about my father's death in my early twenties. My great-aunt, with whom I was very close, shared the story with me, as well as some carefully saved, yellowed newspaper clippings detailing the events from that evening.

I don't remember anything from that night. However, I do know his death sent our family into a tailspin. As a young, fit man, he had not prepared for death. Nothing was in place. No wills. No money. No life insurance. Nothing. To add to the stress, shortly after my father's death we lost our home. You see, the farm was leased; my mother could neither afford nor maintain the property, so we had to leave.

Sometimes, I try to put myself in my mother's shoes. I can't imagine... Suddenly becoming a widow, carrying the weight of the grief, loss, and trauma (I assume, although she never talked about it), being responsible for two small children, having no money, and being completely displaced.

After my father's funeral, discussions began about our options and next steps, which included placing my brother and me in a Children's Home. Thankfully, my godfather stepped up and offered to take us in. It was settled. We were packed up and off we went to live with him in southeast England. Being welcomed into this lovely, warm, kind family was a blessing I will forever be grateful for.

My mum worked hard to support us. Back then, more than 50 years ago, it was tough for women in the work force. Low pay. Long hours. Limited opportunities. I remember her taking the train back and forth to London, arriving home late, exhausted, falling asleep in the chair, and getting up early the next day to leave for the station again. Needless to say, we didn't see her very much.

Adding two small children into a busy, active family of five (two adults, three children) was, I'm sure, a lot. Consequently, this arrangement was temporary, a steppingstone, somewhere to land, while my mum found her feet again. I don't recall how long we stayed with our cousins before it was time to move on again. This time we were off to live with my other godfather and his wife who ran a pub in southern England. This was a more permanent arrangement, with the adults devising a mutually agreeable plan. We had a home, my mum continued to travel back and forth to London, and she helped in the pub on the weekends.

Nestled in the heart of the English countryside, this quintessential village adorned with Tudor architecture and roots extending all the way back to the Middle Ages, became a safe haven for my brother and me. We went to school, made friends, played outside, and enjoyed lots of freedom. Everything was in walking or biking distance. The stream. The playground. The pool. The sweet shop. Slowly our family began to stabilize and heal. This continued for several years. We were happy, well cared for, and our sense of family, belonging, and connection began to sprout again. Life was good.

Fast forward a few years: I was then probably late elementary school age when my mum met a man who was a regular at the pub. Like many relationships, things appeared to be fine at first. He seemed like a nice enough man. Their relationship blossomed to the point of wanting to live together.

I don't remember much discussion—or frankly, choice—before being told we were moving. Oh, and this gentleman had a massive drinking problem. As a result, life for my brother and me went downhill fast. Money problems. Conflict. Chaos. My saving grace was that we were still in close proximity to my home village. Friends' houses and being outdoors became my escape, my safe places. This continued for a couple years.

My mother, a writer by trade, was the bread winner. In search of a better opportunity, she took a job in a different part of the country. Another move, this time far away from the warmth, safety, and familiarity of that little village, which, even now, I consider home. We relocated. The prospect of a new school (at the age of 13) and being away from family and friends was devastating. Needless to say, I was not a happy camper.

I didn't think things could get much worse, yet they did... Our family disintegrated fast. His addiction worsened. He lost his driving privileges and gainful employment became sporadic, which put even more responsibility on my mum's plate.

My teens were tumultuous. I hated the addiction, which I expressed loud and clear. As the stress and conflict increased, mostly between me and my mum's partner, I ran away, skipped school, snuck out of the house, and broke all the rules. The stress in the house was palpable. Today, when I look back, I laugh: I honestly don't know how I graduated high school, wasn't arrested, or worse.

Anyway, the chaos continued...

Fast forward again, to about 16 years old. My family (Mum, brother, and partner) took a trip "back home" to visit my great-aunt, whom I loved very much. Generally, I would jump at the chance of going back to see friends and family; however, relationships were tense. I could not imagine enduring several hours in the car and everything that came along with it, so I begged to stay home. My wish was granted. My first night of freedom. After waving goodbye and closing the front door, I still remember a blanket of peace settling over the house. Quiet and still (something I still cherish today). Finally, there was space to think and feel...

In the middle of the night, I woke to pounding on the door and the phone ringing in the kitchen. Groggy and confused, I plodded downstairs and opened the door to be greeted by two police officers—a man and a woman—who tell me that my mother had just been killed in a car accident.

There was no explanation... No other car was involved. No random objects in the road. No bad weather. No reason to have this accident—other than intoxication.

My brother was thrown from the car. He landed way down the road, badly injured, and close to death. My mother, according to the coroner, died on impact. The driver, her partner, walked away without a scratch. As you can imagine, this put me— and our family—into complete turmoil. A slide into depths no child should have to go.

On the plus side, this time I was older and I had

a well-fashioned defiant streak, which, at the time, served me well.

My brother had a long road ahead of him, with several months of physical healing and reha-bilitation, not to mention coping with the resulting grief, loss, and trauma. The home situation worsened. Within a month or so of the funeral my mum's partner hooked up with another woman, and promptly moved her in. What was bad became a nightmare. I left home.

As you can imagine, I was pretty lost... Thankfully, when I started my journey as an ill-equipped 16-year-old, there was another family locally I could lean on. While I am simplifying things a bit, and not delving into the many details between here and there, I can say that was when I began to realize that there's a big wide world out there.

After leaving home, in an attempt to find my feet and figure out this mess called life, I started to explore, travel, and adventure. I spent time in Greece, Spain, France, and North Africa, and lived in the Canary Islands for a year. This was when a lot of the grief, loss, and anger began bubbling to the surface.

Although I appreciated the beauty of it all—the sea, the colors, the lovely vibrant Spanish culture—there was no real connection. No solace. Nothing like the way I experience the natural world today. Back then, I was just trying to make it through the day... In survival mode, I guess.

After the Canary Islands, there was a quick stint back in England, then off to the United States for the summer. I had heard there was work in the Martha's Vineyard area. "What the heck, let's check it out," was my thinking. With flights booked and a suitcase packed, a friend and I landed in New York City. The summer work we had hoped for had fallen through, and we considered, "Okay, what now?" I had some friends from high school in Los Angeles, California, so we hopped on a Greyhound bus and traveled across the country. It was an amazing experience!

When I think about that trip, I laugh; it seemed like we stopped in the bad end of every single town. I'll never forget the smell of the chemical toilet in the back of the bus and the people we met along the way. All sorts of people. So much diversity, which was lovely.

I stayed with my high school friends for a while. With funds starting to run low, I found a job. I loved California and the outdoor lifestyle. The dry air. The beach and the mountains. Slowly, I began feeling grounded again...

The weeks quickly turned into months, and the months tumbled into years. Although, my high school performance was dismal, I love to read and was fascinated with human behavior (no surprise there...). I decided to enroll in classes at the local community college in Santa Monica. I took a keen interest, kept up with the work, and—for the first time in my life—got decent grades.

By this point, I was running and hiking on a regular basis. Did I mention that I loved being outdoors? The sun. The colors. The ocean. The dry heat. Although, at the time I was enamored with it all, I wasn't cognizant of my connection and the importance of nature in my life.

In my mid-20s, I transferred from community college to the University of California, Los Angeles (UCLA) to start a bachelor's degree in Psychology. I was working and going to school. I had stable housing, friends, and a sense of purpose.

It was around this time that I met and started dating my now husband, who was originally from the Midwest. We had a spark and things between us started getting serious.

To give you the abbreviated version, we dated for a while, with some long-distance stints, back and forth between California and the Midwest. Eventually, after some deaths in his family, we decided to pack up, head back, and give the Midwest a try. Fairly quickly we started a family and built a home. We had a girl, then a boy.

With a family, two small children, grad school, and working part-time, life was in full swing. When my son was either two or three years old (I am terrible with times and dates), I began experiencing some funky physical symptoms in my body.

Stiffness. Swelling. Discomfort. To which, in all the hustle and bustle of life, I paid no attention. Or at least, I tried to ignore, until I literally woke up one morning and couldn't move.

It came on so fast... seemingly overnight. I was getting stiffer and stiffer. By the end of the day, my feet and ankles were so swollen, they would bulge out of my shoes. My fingers resembled little fat sausages. I couldn't wear my wedding ring, turn on a tap, or fasten my bra. Buttons were impossible. Yet, I still had this internship to complete, little humans to care for, and end of term papers to write. I had to figure out what the heck was going on with my body.

After a visit to the doctor, a myriad of blood tests, and a battery of x-rays, I was diagnosed with aggressive rheumatoid arthritis (RA). RA is an autoimmune disorder where your body—the immune system—launches an attack on the joints. I was started on the standard course of care; the RA wasn't responding as hoped. They upped the level of care, which meant infusions of medicine at home, once a week initially, then monthly to see if that would get the RA under control.

I had a horrible reaction after the first dose. I now joke, "I think I must have been allergic to the mouse poop." (Somewhere, along the way, I heard that mouse feces were one of the active ingredients. Don't quote me on that...) Regardless, clearly, the most aggressive treatment was not going to be an option for me.

Back to the rheumatologist to discuss my limited treatment options...

Receiving a diagnosis like this in your late 30s is, frankly, terrifying. My imagination served me a constant stream of images with people—mostly me— wheelchair bound, hunched over with gnarled, knotted fingers and claw-like hands, unable to move, let alone walk or run or hike.

I have a vivid memory of leaving the doctor's office that day. It was one of those beautiful, bright, crisp, Midwestern days. As I walked to the car from that red brick building, a part of me announced loud and clear, "Man, I am not going down that road. This is NOT going to be me." From that moment, it seemed like my whole being—mind, body, and spirit—committed to being the poster child for recovering from RA.

I went back on the standard dose of daily medication and got super serious about my health, starting with food, exercise, and a scramble for effective coping strategies. Although my life was stable, a big part of me was still in survival mode. The changes and all the stress coupled with buckets of unresolved grief, loss, and trauma were under the surface screaming, "Take care of me..."

None of that childhood crap had been dealt with. I just kept going and going and going (like the

Energizer bunny). I now know that my body was sending me signs and signals, trying—urging me to slow down and take care of myself.

My diet had been horrible for years. I was eating a lot of processed foods, carbs, and sugar, sugar, sugar like crazy. Boxes of cookies, cakes, and chocolate bars. All packed with highly refined, unpronounceable lists of ingredients. Although I would run now and again, healthy movement and time outdoors were sporadic. Like an ostrich with its head in the sand, there was no connection with nature. No wonder. No awe. Nothing. Physically, mentally, spiritually I was not in a good place. My body was screaming, "Slow down!"

Thanks to the RA, I finally heard the message loud and clear. I started taking my health seriously and my healing journey began...

*Please share a little about the role of nature in your healing process.*

After the diagnosis, I took a long, hard look at my life and began to consider what I needed and didn't need. Starting with food, I stripped out all the processed food. Basically, if it came in a box, I didn't eat it. I added lots of water, fruits, veggies, and grains into my daily diet. By that point, I wasn't a red meat eater. I did eat chicken and fish, which I was fine to continue for a while. Through my education I was beginning to understand the mind, and be fascinated by the mind/body connection, so I added meditation and yoga to my week. At the time, I was also learning about psychoimmunology (the study of interactions between the mind, the nervous system, the immune system, and health). I focused on healing imagery. I imagined lots of little Pac-Man characters, munching their way through my system, consuming all the inflammation around my joints. While chronic fatigue often accompanies RA, as the swelling and stiffness began to ease up, I felt more energetic. So much so, that I was back to running more regularly. Slowly, over time, I began feeling a bit better.

Up to this point, I had been a road runner: pounding on pavement and sidewalks, looking down at my feet, interested in little more than getting the job done. A friend suggested I try trail running. After the initial, "Are you kidding?" reaction, I was curious. We would lace up, sometimes once or twice a week, head out and hit the trails. That experience was a game changer. Getting out into those woods, among the trees, with the birds, and the peace and quiet—it became my solace.

Here I was, in my mid-40s, out on the trail in the safety of the woods and trees, when my body decided it was time to begin letting go of some of the grief. There was no intention, no grand plan—the layers of loss just began melting away. I remember certain areas of the woods—deep in the quiet, soft, majestic pines—which seemed to magically unlock waves and waves of grief. I could feel knots and surges of it coming up through my body. There were physical sensations, literally pain in my heart, chest, and gut—sometimes it would be so intense, it would take my breath away causing me to gasp for air. This out-of-breath feeling, was a completely new sensation. The emotions poured out of me. Hot tears flowed down my face, some filled with rage, some with a mixture of hurt and deep sadness. Then, as if wrapped in a warm, loving embrace, a sense of calm would settle over my body and mind. This happened over and over again: the more I ran, the more grief I shed.

My body responded well. With improved nutrition, guided imagery, and the trail running, I started feeling even better: physically fitter, mentally stronger, and emotionally lighter. What's more, the inflammation markers began decreasing. Day-to-day, I was able to do mostly what I wanted. With the green light from the doctor, we started decreasing the medication.

I was getting out into nature a lot... Although I was having these significant experiences, I still didn't fully realize the power of nature and the natural world. Yes, I'm out there. Yes, I'm on the planet. Yes, I'm in the woods. Yet I still didn't feel the deep, deep connection that I feel currently.

Today, for me, being out in nature is best described as a full body experience—akin to a flow state or metaphysical experience. It's mind. It's body. It's spirit. It's the exchange of oxygen between me and the plants and the trees. It's feeling deeply rooted in the ground beneath my feet. It's the wind. It's the sound of the birds. It's the light, the rain, the sun, the moon. It's being out there *with* the planet. I could go on and on...

This deep connection with the natural world didn't fully kick in until I started backpacking. Yes, trail running was a huge step, and I love hiking; however, backpacking took being out in nature to a whole other level.

As I connected more with the trail running/hiking community, I wanted to test myself—do longer, harder hikes and experience the "back-country" I was hearing so much about. I bought myself a backpack to celebrate my 55th birthday and signed-up for a three-day, two-night back-packing trip and had an absolute blast. I loved every messy, buggy, uncomfortable moment of it!

I haven't looked back. This experience deepened my connection with nature and sparked my passion for the natural world. Since then, I've done plenty of backpacking, learned a lot about myself, and had some amazing adventures along the way.

In the last five years, my connection—relationship—with the natural world has become a cornerstone of my daily life. If I go two or three days without being in the woods or among trees, I begin to feel it in my mind and body. Nature feeds my soul in countless ways.

Sitting under a tree or by a creek, meditating, connecting with the earth and the vastness of it all and realizing that I am a tiny, integral part of it all helps me gain perspective. In the past there was a lot of confusion, anger, loss, despair, and loneliness. Through nature, running, and therapy—a lot of therapy—I have worked through much of that. Time out in the natural world has been, and continues to be, an important part of my sanity.

*Is there an experience in nature that stands out in your mind as particularly powerful?*

There are so many... I'm going to go back to backpacking because many of those experiences have been profound. Everything from waking up in the mountains on a cool misty morning, where the moment is so still and quiet. When the sound of my tent unzipping is the only noise that breaks the silence. I head up to the ridge to catch the first rays of the day, the warmth of the little tin cup of tea heats my hands, sitting there among the wonder and majesty of it all. Every time I'm out there, there's always something new. I love the sunrise and sunset. It's an honor and a great day—regardless of where I am—if I get to experience both these wonders in the same day. I also love knowing that every time I drive to the trail head, put on my pack, and step out on that trail there will be something new to learn or discover or experience.

As for the seasons, I love the summertime. I love the springtime. I love the autumn and I'm learning to love the winter. This has taken me a while, since I am not a fan of the cold. That said, I'm learning to celebrate and embrace the beauty, the spirit, and the importance of winter.

When I am out in nature, I feel grounded, present, my body feels clear, my mind feels sharp. I feel at home. Creative energy flows through me. Sometimes, I simply walk along—breathe in, breathe out—just soaking everything in. Other times, I am focused and intentional about really noticing. Literally noticing shapes, colors, trees, deeply looking at leaves, butterflies, the crags in the bark—whatever is in my view. Minimal thought. No judgement. I encourage you to try it—it's a neat experience.

Other times it's that feeling I get when I come up to a vista. Sometimes there's so much emotion, right? You work really hard to get up the mountain or climb to this elevation, and you come around the corner to be greeted by views that take your breath away. This was especially prevalent for me in the White Mountains of New Hampshire.

For me, witnessing the peaks or vistas or valleys inspire complete awe. Sometimes, even today, when I feel the majesty, the wonder, the connection with something much larger—tears come and a sense of peace settles deep into my bones. What else has the power to do that?

Trust me, connecting with nature does not have to involve some grand trip. It's also simple everyday things... I remember being up on a ledge in a local park, getting caught in a thunderstorm, and having to hunker down to wait for the storm to pass. That was an awesome experience.

Camping, all cozy in my little tent, and the smell of the campfire. Setting up my tent so I know I'll wake up to the sunrise. Enjoying and exploring the night sky. Hearing little hints of scratching outside the tent, as I hope little critters aren't getting into my pack. Things like this—big and small—opportunities for connection and wonder—are limitless.

I love filtering water from streams. There are many places I've been where you have to carry and filter water as you go. I love that! Stopping, taking off my pack, setting up the filter, drawing up the water. Filtering water makes you stop. Slow down. Notice. Right by the edge of the creek looking for just the right spot. It takes time and care to collect water. I enjoy looking up and realizing—seeing—that I am in the midst of it all. The water cycle, the life cycle, the reciprocal relationship is wonderful. I love the mess, the bugs, the sweat, being dirty or stinky or whatever. In those moments I feel gratitude for all that.

I also love coming home, hugging my husband, seeing my family, taking a hot shower, and crawling into my cozy bed. I am grateful for this too. Together, all these experiences have enriched my life and mended my soul...

*What would you tell people who are currently experiencing what you went through?*

I want people to know two things: it can get better and it's never too late. Like I said earlier, as I head into the final quarter of my life, I'm in a much, much better place. I am probably healthier, and in better shape—mentally, physically, spiritually—than I have ever been. The RA is in remission, and I am completely medication free!

I encourage patience. I would say, "Keep trying." Keep trying to find what works for you. Trust me, great doctors and powerful medicine have been an important part of my journey. I am thankful for those things. And, also, trust that you know yourself best... You are the expert on you. I encourage people to reflect inward and try to connect with those healing parts or healing wisdom that know what's best for you.

I believe we all have a wise internal wisdom or healer. For me, getting in touch with that part of my self was crucial. I also believe that the natural world, combined with movement, provides a powerful elixir. Being outside, being in the trees, being on the water, being active, moving the body, breathing in fresh air, and soaking up sunlight are all parts of the healing process. Along with simple things like drinking enough water, eating fruits, vegetables, beans, grains—all things Mother Nature so generously provides for us.

Mindfulness, meditation, and therapy have been invaluable, particularly in working through some of my childhood traumas. I still see a therapist: she's an important part of my team. I am far from "better"—the healing and discovery process is life-long.

Honesty, with yourself and others, is also important. Being truthful about the challenges, about the loss, the grief, and the pain. Being candid at this point in your life—about what you're willing to do and what you're not willing to do—and then setting boundaries accordingly is essential. There are certain things I'm just not willing to do anymore and there are certain things I have to do... So, I make time to be outside. I make time to hike. I make time to backpack. I make time to meditate.

I run a business and I'm a writer. I have a family, a grandchild, and even though my children are grown and we are close-knit, they still have needs. I work my "care time" into my schedule. Planning, compromise, communication, and boundaries help me balance my time. It's all about balance: balancing life and time and listening to the mind and the body and the natural world around you.

*What other tools have been helpful during your healing process?*

I read a lot... You will find many of my favorite books listed under Resources. I love podcasts too; they have been so helpful. In fact, in the spirit of giving back—and hopefully helping others—I am launching a podcast called *Living Big Mindfully* (see Resources for links).

People want to find a fix: it's like they see themselves as broken, and consequently, in search— or need—of something out there; something outside themselves to "fix" them. You know what I mean: this thing, that thing, this program, that pill or product, blah, blah, blah. Honestly, in my humble opinion, that's all hype and hogwash. Why? Well, first we— *you*—are not broken. Yes, there may be things we need to work on, uncover, discover, and work through—this is a natural part of being human. We all have "stuff." We are humans with messy, complicated lives, *and* we are equipped, naturally, with an incredible array of resources—internally and externally—designed for healing. No "fixing" needed!

I believe that we have to start with ourselves: that the journey begins on the inside and the answers come from within. Getting clear about what you want, what you need, what you're willing to do, and what you're unwilling to do is a good starting point.

Although not often discussed, massage can also be a powerful part of the healing process. At the time of writing there is limited research about the role of massage in the treatment of grief, loss, and trauma. However, I can personally attest to the benefits of regular massage with a skilled, appropriately licensed practitioner.

Our bodies soak up the shocks, losses, frustrations, and the traumas of everyday life (past and present). These "memories" get stored quietly away—often for decades—suspended in time, held in the tissue, the cells, the muscles, the fascia, manifesting as tightness, tension, tingling, or other physical sensations.

As I began processing the grief and loss, my left shoulder developed odd numb, tingling sensations that would flare up at night. The discomfort would shoot down my arm, causing restlessness and sleep disturbance. Intuitively, I had a sense that this was stuff from old issues that had been unconsciously locked away in my body for decades. The massage therapist and I worked on my neck, shoulder, upper arm, and back. As she dug into that area, it felt like years of tension were being released at a cellular level. I remember laughing because it literally "hurt so good." After those sessions, I felt absolutely drained, beaten up, and wiped out.

Is my experience so surprising? Probably not... Psychiatrist Bessel van der Kolk, MD in his book *The Body Keeps the Score: Brain, Mind and Body in the Healing of Trauma* talks about the way "memory of helplessness is stored as muscle tension or feelings" in the body. Additionally, in her article *Letting it Go: A Transformative Session of Massage Therapy* (2020), massage therapist Amanda Brauman King shares her thoughts about, "How wonderful [it is] to let go of grief, anguish, anger, frustration, humiliation or whatever else our loyal tissues may have packaged up in literal human Ziplocs." Her eloquent description offers further support for the role of massage in the healing process. What was the outcome for me? My shoulder issue fully resolved in about three sessions.

Building a team I like and trust has been important. Take the time to find the right therapist, doctor, chiropractor, meditation teacher, yoga instructor, etc. Don't stick with a provider that's not working for or with you. If you're not feeling heard, understood, and cared for find someone else. I have a three-session rule, I tell my clients this too… Try a provider three times; if you're not feeling it, then move on. Keep exploring until you find a good fit. I went through several rheumatologists before I found a woman whom I felt was on the same page. She "got" me, she listened, and she supported my desire for a full recovery or "spontaneous remission," as the medical profession likes to call it.

*From surviving to thriving: Tell me a bit about your life today.*

At this point in my life, I don't look back much. Everything that happened to me, even the difficult stuff has, in some way, informed my life. I am where I am today because of—or maybe even in spite of—it all.

Nature has played a huge role in my healing and, frankly, spiritual journey. Now, when I am out in nature, in the natural world, that time is special. I try to savor it. That's when I connect with my higher power, when I give and receive offerings, reflect, and express gratitude. Again, these experiences can range from a few moments sitting in a sunny window, to a walk around the block, to a longer hike or bike ride.

For me, a vital part of thriving—healing—has been working on getting that grief out of my body. Stuff gets stuck in the body, stuck in the gut, stuck in the chest. The muscles. The cells. The very fabric of our being. Grief, trauma, loss is held in the body, as much as it is held in the mind and memories. There is a strong body of evidence that's beginning to connect unresolved grief, trauma, and chronic stress to autoimmune disorders and even cancer. Effective healing is a holistic process—it happens on many levels. Mind. Body. Spirit.

In my case, with no genetic disposition, I believe this to be true. I had a lot of unresolved grief, loss, and trauma—and like layers of stubborn sediment, it built up over the years and came out through my body. As I worked through the trauma—mentally and physically—and made other changes in my life (food, movement, time out in nature) I got better. I have been in complete remission from the autoimmune disorder for several years—which I'm so very thankful for.

I work hard to stay healthy. One of my biggest fears is being bedridden and unable to move—the irony of developing a condition that tugs on that fear is not lost on me. So, I do some sort of movement/exercise every day. Sometimes it's a run or a longer hike, sometimes it's a seven-day backpacking adventure, sometimes it's a 20-minute walk down the road and back. That movement piece is vital. I also mix in stretching, meditation, and weight training.

The stretching is important for flexibility, balance, and connecting with the body, mind, and breath. Mindfulness/meditation—another mind/body/soul connection—comes and goes. Sometimes it's 20 minutes every day, other days it's a bit choppy—five minutes here and there. At this point in my life, any small moment is an opportunity to be mindful. When I wake up, I have a routine, a ritual, if you like. I make my bed, I have tea, I sit and notice the day. Maybe the sunrise, maybe the mist, maybe the birdsong, maybe the light. I sit and breathe, soaking it all in. I'll also connect inside myself—add a body scan of sorts, checking in with my parts, my mood, and my energy. That's my quiet contemplative time. Then I'm ready to get my day rolling.

Even walking from the car into the office presents an opportunity... I am fortunate to rent a beautiful office space. The building is surrounded by trees and there's a wonderful little creek that flows by, within earshot. Sometimes it's gushing, sometimes it's a soft trickle there's always a lot of birds and bird activity. So, in the few steps it takes to walk from the car to the front door, I use those moments to take a few breaths, to connect with the earth. I look up at the big sky, and just notice the natural world around me.

When you think about it, there are so many moments, right? People often think that connecting with nature must be planned or somehow squeezed into a weekend or vacation. I am learning—and here to tell you—that that's just not so.

For at least three years I have been trying to grow sunflowers. After many fruitless, lackluster attempts, this summer I have managed to raise a beautiful crop of sunflowers, which I am so excited about. I say "raise" for a reason... This year I have felt or developed a different—more reciprocal—relationship with the earth, gardening, and growing. From preparing the soil, to planting the seeds, to watching, waiting, and wondering if anything will sprout. Watering the little green shoots in the evening. Watching them grow, wondering at the marvel of it...

For the first time in my life, I felt a care for nature—like a mother tending her children. Admiring all those little heads, eager for the budding blooms to show their potential. Share their glory with the world. Have you ever noticed the amazing patterns of little sunflower buds? They have this incredible complex fractal pattern... Did you know sunflower buds follow the arc of the sun? In the morning, their heads face the east, as if they are patiently waiting to celebrate the sunrise. At mid-day, their heads are up straight, standing at attention, like proud pencils in a pencil box. When the sun sets, their heads orient toward the west, as if they are honoring and aware that another precious day has ended. I didn't know or feel any of this prior to this year.

The last five years have been an incredible journey in many ways. Connecting in big and small ways with the planet, Mother Earth, and the natural world, not to mention the love and care I have discovered through gardening (I have never been a gardener; I could hardly keep a cactus alive).

This season the sunflowers are thriving. I have also, for the first time grown lettuce and we have jalapeños, strawberries, and little baby tomatoes arriving. I share these experiences to offer a glimpse of what opening to nature can feel like and, hopefully, inspire or spark thoughts about what might be possible for you.

Being open to this kind of give and take, the gratitude, this respect, the understanding that we are all interconnected with the natural world, our planet, this ecosystem feels peaceful, like I now know how to live my best life. Furthermore, I believe, that when we are rooted or connected in some way with this wonderful planet, we can all begin to heal and thrive.

I feel fortunate... I love my work. As you know, I am an author and a writer, and connecting with real people and sharing their inspirational stories gives me a great deal of pleasure. It's also another way I can give back. My hope is that something in one of these stories will spark something in you—there's that reciprocal relationship again. That inter-connectedness. Which, I might add, is the opposite of disconnectedness, loneliness, and isolation; such a painful place to be. I've been there and know firsthand what that feels like. Feeling connected with Mother Nature, like I'm a tiny part of it all, has profoundly changed my life.

### *If you had one piece of sage advice to offer, what would it be?*

Hmm, sage advice... I would reiterate the importance of patience and not giving up. Yes, keep trying, be patient, and never give up. As long as we are breathing, we can make changes. Read, learn, connect with nature, build your healing team, and remember, it's never too late to begin the healing process.

*Is there anything you want to add that we didn't cover?*

Trust me, my life is far from perfect and there are still times when I feel the sting of the loss—particularly around Mother's Day and Christmas. I mentioned earlier that this last quarter of my life (so far) has been more pleasant—better—in comparison to the first quarter. Of course, back then, I had no idea what I was going to do or where I would be. I could not have predicted how my life looks today. Evidence that our past neither defines us nor determines our future.

I have come to view the world and our human nature as limitless. We think we are sure about so much, when in reality, we know very little—a fraction about the brain, a little bit about the nervous system, the body, and how we work in relationship with the natural world. One great example is circadian rhythms—natural processes that affect all living things (even sunflowers). It takes courage to face your demons. I have a lot of compassion for people who are working on healing—it's not easy. If you are struggling right now with anything—addiction, depression, anxiety, a physical health concern, an autoimmune disorder—I encourage you to connect with some like-minded, supportive people, and try to get outside and move—even a little bit. And remember, you are not alone...

———

# LISA SMITH

Backpacker—healing alcoholism and trauma—rebuilding her life
through Twelve-Step programs and hiking the Pacific Crest Trail

*"...I was so sick. I remember lying in the
bathtub with the shower on throwing up, just
like I had a thousand times before. Somewhere,
deep inside a part of me was saying, 'Enough is
enough. [I] cannot do this anymore.'"*

– Lisa Smith

**WHAT STRUCK ME** about my conversation with Lisa
was her openness, energy, and true zest for life.
What an inspiration! Incredible when you consider
where she was with an out-of-control addiction.

Lisa takes us through her very real roller coaster
ride with alcohol, bravely narrating the highs, the
lows, the loss, and the trauma—truths that often go
hand-in-hand with chronic, active addiction.

Lisa also recounts the details of her personal
road to recovery, which included the decision to
hike the Pacific Crest Trail (PCT) from end to
end—a whopping 2650 miles! Subsequently, she
found herself completely rebuilding her mental,
physical, and spiritual health. Lisa generously
shares her story in the spirit, and with the hope of

helping other people reclaim their lives. She is proof that—on the other side of addiction—a rich, full life is possible.

The fact is that addiction is a debilitating condition that affects hundreds of millions of people throughout the world. As a mother, a clinician, and a woman whose life has been deeply affected by the devastation of addiction, my heart was deeply touched by Lisa's story. I hope it will touch yours too. Thank you, Lisa, for sharing and shining some of your light, love, and hope into the world—you are truly an inspiration!


## Lisa S

*Tell me a bit about you and your background.*

My father was in forestry well before I was born. He was comfortable working and living in the outdoors. My mom, not so much. Of course, she went along with the camping trips, as long as they weren't too rustic. As a child I remember my family building a cabin which meant a lot of time outside, in nature, playing, and entertaining myself.

Probably because of those early experiences I am very comfortable in and around nature. I love being in the mountains and the forests. I have memories of being quite small, playing in the woods, alone for hours and hours, making mud pies and climbing trees. I wasn't afraid of animals, or worried about getting dirty, or scared of anything really. I felt comfortable out there.

I have a twin brother who is extremely athletic and capable. As a child, I felt like I could never compete with him. Consequently, I avoided anything outdoors that felt competitive. I think that's one reason I really loved unstructured time outside. If I got a hint of athletic competition or a sense that something required a lot of physical skill, I quickly felt intimidated and shied away. Things changed as I moved into adulthood.

*Diving into the tough topic, tell me a bit about your personal journey/experience.*

Growing up, there was a lot of drinking, and probably alcoholism, in my family. Unfortunately, the apple didn't fall far from the tree. In hindsight, I was probably an alcoholic from the first time I had a drink. I remember that experience like it was yesterday.

I was 11, maybe 12. We were at my grandmother's house celebrating her birthday when one of my aunts thought it would be hilarious to feed me drinks. To this day, I remember the rush of the alcohol and feeling like I could not get enough. I wanted more and more. I remember going around the party sneaking the adults' drinks when they weren't looking and consuming as much as I possibly could. I don't actually remember this; however, I was told that I—a child—stood in the middle of the party and chugged a beer in front of everyone. Apparently, I passed out and woke up the next day feeling absolutely mortified.

Paradoxically, I also recall feeling exhilarated and thinking, "That was amazing. I loved that, but just don't get so drunk next time." I was 11 or 12 years old! Right there, in that moment that became my life's mission—to chase that feeling—but not get quite so out of control. That was the beginning of my journey with addiction.

As a teenager, things got worse: I was blacking out and making a fool of myself at parties with friends. I remember trying to quit drinking for the first time when I was 16 years old. Clearly, needing to stop drinking at 16 was a huge red flag for alcoholism. I tried so hard to control it. Yet, I kept the love affair going.

I knew there was a lot of untreated alcoholism in my family. I just didn't see myself as having a problem, partly because I was trying so hard to control it. I thought, "I can't be an alcoholic because I am trying hard. People who were real alcoholics don't try…"

I tried all sorts of tricks in an attempt to calibrate the amount I drank. My goal was to enjoy drinking, without the embarrassment of getting too drunk. Sometimes that worked; most of the time it didn't. Somehow, I managed to keep a lid on it, functioning well, for many years. I graduated high school, completed two university degrees, and created a decent life for myself. However, over time, alcohol became more and more dominant in my life. It took up so much of my mental space and energy. Plus, due to the drinking, I found myself in a lot of uncomfortable, embarrassing, and frankly dangerous situations. No one knew...

I vividly remember one example of how hard I was trying to control my drinking. I was out one evening with friends who were social drinkers. I was determined to pace myself. I decided to copy exactly what they did. I ordered the same drink and only took a sip when they did. I watched the level in their glasses. They took a sip, I took a sip. To slow down my consumption to a "normal" level was absolute torture for me. I couldn't fathom how or why anyone would drink so slowly. I could not relax, let alone have a good time. My brain was obsessed with trying to figure out, "When is the next sip coming?" What's more—even with all of this—I still didn't consider myself as having a problem with alcohol.

This pattern continued throughout my late teens and 20s. In my early 30s, my health began declining and I started feeling like crap. I was having severe unexplained allergic reactions to pretty much everything. I went to a naturopath who recommended an elimination diet. No sugar. No caffeine. No alcohol.

I took her advice. Boy, I got so sick. The naturopath felt the sickness was due to all the toxins leaving my body. I realize, now, that I was withdrawing from alcohol. I literally spent three days in bed. At the time, it didn't cross my mind that I was in acute alcohol withdrawal. Now, I know that it can be dangerous— sometimes fatal—to stop drinking cold turkey.

Regardless, that wasn't enough to stop me. The cycle quickly continued. I would drink heavily with periods of being totally out of control. Then, I would swear off alcohol forever. That would last for a day or two. Then I'd be right back into full swing again.

A pivotal moment came in my mid-30s. One evening, I decided to go out with friends for a glass of wine. I told myself, "Okay, only one glass." I had it all planned out, with all the usual safeguards in place (a certain amount of money and only one credit card). I really didn't want to make a fool out of myself or get into trouble—again. I ordered my glass of wine. Before I knew it, I was on to the next glass, and then the next. I just kept ordering drink after drink. It wasn't unusual for my friends, after a couple of glasses of wine, to leave the bar and head home. It makes sense, they had had enough. It was time to go... That night I pretended to leave with them, and then headed right back to the bar. That was typical of me. Of course, I'd make all sorts of "new friends" and, consequently, end up in some terrible situations.

To this day, I don't actually know what happened that night. I do know I ended up blacked out—unconscious—in a police cell. When I came to, I had no idea where I was or how I got there. I do remember waking up and looking down at my hands to see if I had blood on them. I honestly didn't know... Had I killed someone? Had I been in a fight? Was there a car wreck? It was the most terrifying feeling I've ever had.

I realize now that I was being held in the drunk tank at the local jail because I was so intoxicated. It was horrible. I was terrified. The shame. The humiliation. It was the most awful feeling I've ever had in my life.

Once I sobered up, I was allowed a phone call. I called a family friend, who picked me up from jail and took me home. I was so sick. I remember lying in the bathtub with the shower on, throwing up—just like I had a thousand times before. This time, somewhere, deep inside a part of me was saying, "Enough is enough. You cannot do this anymore." Even with all of this, as ridiculous as this sounds, another part of me couldn't fathom the thought of actually quitting—stopping drinking for good. Once again, my brain assured me that, "I just had to figure out how to stop getting so drunk."

My plan was to go to an Alcoholics Anonymous (AA) meeting. Not because I thought that they could help me stop drinking. Again, that didn't occur to me, which, in hindsight seems crazy. I honestly didn't know that people who drank like me successfully stopped drinking. I had never known or seen anyone who was an alcoholic stop drinking. I thought AA was a support group for people who couldn't quit drinking. I thought if I went there, I would see all these "miserable pathetic losers" and that would scare me into drinking normally. This was my grand plan.

The same day I woke up in jail, I found a meeting. I sat outside, in my car, for 20 minutes before going in. I was petrified, mortified, and full of shame. To my surprise (of course...), instead of a bunch of losers and people who were miserable, I found amazing people from all walks of life who were sober! Furthermore, people were happy and full of hope, laughing, and sharing their stories. People who once drank like I was drinking.

Right there, in that moment, I felt a glimmer of hope. Maybe it was actually possible to stop drinking! Yet, I still couldn't imagine the thought of my entire life without drinking; it all seemed way too daunting. I remember hearing someone say, "Don't worry about having a life without drinking, just see if you can get to bedtime tonight without having a drink. Then come back tomorrow." I was like, "Okay, maybe I'll try that. I'll try making it to bedtime. I'm fairly sure I can do that. Then I will go back tomorrow." That's exactly what I did. I made it until bedtime without a drink and went to a meeting the next day. Again and again, a day at a time, I tried to make it until bedtime without having a drink, then went to a meeting the following day. I did that over and over. Sometimes I went to three meetings a day—whatever it took—until I could begin to string some sober time together and begin to function again.

People in recovery talk a lot about "one day at a time." For me, in those early days of sobriety, it was more like living one hour at a time. Working to overcome the physical withdrawals and the mountain of shame and guilt and humiliation was the beginning of my recovery journey. After a while, I started to get my feet under me.

Because I had been drinking heavily for so long the withdrawal symptoms were uncomfortable. I constantly felt sick. I had profuse sweating, splitting headaches, the shakes, and I couldn't sleep. Although I work in healthcare, I didn't seek medical help. I was so embarrassed, I could not ask for the help I needed. In hindsight, alcohol withdrawal can be so dangerous. I know that was not a smart choice. Thankfully, once I made it through those first two or three weeks I started feeling—physically—a lot better.

Mentally, however, that was a different story. I was carrying all that shame, loss, and trauma. I kept it all inside. A secret. I kept pushing through; I didn't take any time off work. I convinced myself that I would be completely mortified if anyone found out I had a drinking problem. At times, I remember feeling so raw, as if I were walking through the world completely naked with no ability to cope or protect myself.

I could not understand how I had reached this point. I'm a smart person. I've read all Oprah's self-help books. Without the alcohol it was like I was completely clueless about feelings, mental health, or coping strategies. With the alcohol gone, I found I had no ability to cope with stress. I realized I needed some tools. And I needed them fast.

I'd cry in my car, on my lunch break. I would call someone from AA. They would talk me down. The big focus of AA is finding a higher power. I didn't want anything to do with religion or God. Yet, the people in my AA meetings emphasized, over and over again, the importance of finding spirituality—praying, connecting with something bigger than myself. They encouraged me to consider options outside traditional religion: God. Church. Things like that. I had to find something to connect with spiritually. That's when I began tapping into nature. I started getting outdoors, being by the ocean, being by a tree. I learned I could pray to a tree. A horse. My dog. It didn't matter. I could send prayers out to Mother Earth. I could connect with spirituality in that way. That was something I knew I could do...

*Please share a little about the role of nature in your healing process.*

I am fortunate to have had a background of being in nature in my childhood. For me, being out in nature feels comfortable. I had done a bit of hiking and backpacking when I was in my 20s. I also brought a liter of alcohol on that backpacking trip; crazy to think about that now—it was a five-day trip. I remember my primary concern was running out of alcohol.

Any suggestions to go out for a walk or go for a hike or go and sit by the ocean all felt natural to me. With time, connecting with nature became the one place where I felt okay in the world. Where I felt different. Better. In the regular world, I felt raw and exposed, like I had no skin on. When I was alone in the woods or by the water I felt okay. No one was evaluating me. No one was watching me. No one was judging me. I could begin to be myself.

I don't know if I have the words to describe how powerful nature has been in my healing journey. One of the key elements in recovery is finding a power that is greater than you. Being in nature, and connecting with the natural world again, it soon became obvious that there is a power so much greater than me. Nature helped me restore my sanity.

When you are in front of the mountains or walking through a huge old-growth forest it's easy to imagine something bigger. A vastness. Something powerful. I began to feel, see, and more importantly understand, that I was a small part of the intricate fabric of life. This sense is especially powerful when I am in the forest. The forest is where I feel the most calm and connected, where I'm not worrying about the future or obsessing about the past. This is where I feel present and closest to my higher power.

In nature I can be in the moment. I can use all my senses. I can hear the birds, feel the warmth of the sun on my face, and notice the breeze on my skin. In the early days of recovery, this was vital for me. Nature and the natural world continue to play an important part in my mental and physical health care. Even now, when I am feeling disconnected, discouraged, or overwhelmed, I head out into nature. Fundamentally, I never lost that connection through all the drinking. Even back then, I had aspirations to do more hiking. But, honestly, apart from not being able to carry enough alcohol, I just didn't think I could do it.

Early in my sobriety, as I started spending more and more time in nature, the idea of a longer hike started appealing to me. Off in the distance, I had this pipe dream of—someday—hiking the Pacific Crest National Scenic Trail (PCT). One of the longest footpaths in the United States, the trail stretches 2650 miles (4265 kilometers) all the way from the Mexican border to the Canadian border via California, Oregon, and Washington.

The more my head cleared, the more I started to consider what it might be like to hike the PCT. In preparation, and to test myself, I started out with a couple of longer hikes. They went well. Then I decided to hike the Tour du Mont Blanc in Europe, which is about 106 miles (170 kilometers). That went well. The following year, I hiked the Tahoe Rim Trail, a 170 mile (274 kilometers) loop around the Tahoe Rim Basin which is located in the Sierra Nevada ranges of Nevada and California in the United States.

Frankly, I had no idea what I was capable of; yet somewhere inside I really wanted to try. I've never been especially athletic, and I don't consider myself to be super fit. Regardless, both these longer hikes went well and were good experiences.

In the fall that year, my stepfather, who was in his early 60s, died of a sudden stroke. Once I had recovered from the shock, I started reflecting back over my life—and the reality of life and death hit me. His life was cut short suddenly, without warning. He never got to retire. He never got to live all his dreams. His death woke me up to the fact that time—life—is guaranteed to no one. Including me... If I wanted to do a big hike, I should just go ahead and do it. So, I applied for a permit that November and started hiking the PCT the following April.

By then, I was two and a half years sober. Even with that, I felt nervous about the trek from a recovery point of view. I was worried about leaving my recovery community, my routines, my support systems. Believe it or not, two and a half years is considered quite early in sobriety—early to be undertaking something like this.

I was getting through life pretty well. I wasn't thinking about drinking every day. Overall, I felt fairly solid. I knew that as long as I kept doing the things I needed to do—spiritual practices, prayer, meditation, and staying connected to my recovery community—I would be okay. Every other week or so, I'd find a small town where I would attend 12-step meetings. I'd show up in these tiny little mountain towns. Sometimes, there might be a group of four or five people. Between my spiritual practice, connection with my sponsor, being out in nature, and the meetings, I made it through.

Honestly, drinking didn't occur to me. Because I was spending 100 percent of my time out in nature, I felt so connected to my higher power. Yes, I was malnourished, injured, and my body was wrecked. Yet, my spirit felt so full—drinking was the furthest thing from my mind.

You might be thinking, "Well sure, who's going to be drinking out in the wilderness?" Interestingly, there is a trail culture especially on the longer trails in the United States, of people called Trail Angels. Kind souls who leave things like food and supplies for hikers at the trail heads. It wouldn't be unusual to be walking through the desert and there, literally, in the middle of nowhere would be a cooler full of beer. If I hadn't been in a good place, I know I would have been tempted. Thankfully, it didn't faze me. I knew that picking up one drink was like playing Russian roulette: who knows where I'd end up? In my mind, I always go back to the night I woke up in jail.

*Is there an experience in nature that stands out in your mind as particularly powerful?*

You know, there was a moment on the PCT that stands out to me... It was my second to last day on the trail. The sky was the most brilliant shade of blue, it was just so beautiful. I came up, over a mountain pass when this huge valley opened up in front of me. In that moment, I felt an incredible feeling of freedom sweep over me. I was literally surrounded by endless natural beauty. I felt like I could run and run and run in any direction. I had this voice in my head which said, "This is why you went through all that." For the first time in a very long time, I felt 100 percent free. I'm getting choked-up as I reflect... This is why I had to do all of that—to have freedom: physical freedom, emotional freedom, spiritual freedom, the freedom that comes from being in nature. And, ultimately, the freedom of not being tied to the next drink.

Right then, in that moment, the purpose of this massive endeavor became clear. It was time to truly free myself from all the pain, all the suffering, all those moments of lying in the bottom of my bathtub throwing up. I finally felt free...

### *What would you tell people who are currently experiencing what you went through?*

Great question! I think the biggest lesson I have learned is that "rock bottom" looks different for everyone. I have seen people reach the point where they feel like they just can't go on anymore. When this happens, options present themselves. In my case, I remember thinking about ending my life. Sadly, I know people who have chosen that option. I want people to hear that no matter how bad things seem, there is *always* the option of asking for help. I admit that I am pathologically self-sufficient and independent. Asking for help was the hardest thing I have ever done in my life, particularly at that moment. So, yes, a part of me wishes I would have asked for help sooner, and yet, at the same time, I know that I needed to get to a point of complete desperation—so low—where I felt like I had no other options.

So, what would I tell someone? Please, if you are reading this and struggling with anything—mental health, substance use, physical health concerns—

know that there is help out there (please see Resources for options).

Looking back, I also think it would have been a good idea to get some medical help. Despite working in health care, it didn't cross my mind to get medical assistance for the alcohol withdrawal. Coming off alcohol cold turkey can have serious medical complications. People die from severe alcohol withdrawal. In my mind, I thought that detox was only for withdrawal from drugs like heroin. I encourage people to get the mental and physical help they need. Addiction is a lonely, isolating condition— the more healthy support you have rooting for you the better. I was very fortunate.

I also believe nature can play a big role in the healing and recovery process. The natural world is a part of our fundamental humanness. Being out in nature connects us to our most primitive roots. I would encourage people to try getting outside. It doesn't have to be a massive hike. Try sitting under a tree at your local park, take a walk by a body of water, drive through the countryside with the windows down. Take in the air. Notice how you feel…

*What other tools have been helpful during your healing process?*

It's funny, before facing the truth about my addiction and consequently getting sober, I tried so many things. I got organized. I changed my diet. I started a gratitude practice. I exercised. I even tried hypnosis. Honestly, I credit AA and therapy for changing my life.

A big part of 12-step recovery is about helping others. Now, I sponsor other people on their recovery journeys. Volunteering, giving back, and helping others has been an important part of my healing process, particularly in terms of my emotional and spiritual well-being.

As for books, the famous *Alcoholics Anonymous: The Big Book* saved my life. I picked it up, within a few days I had read it from cover-to-cover. It made so much sense. I found all the answers I was searching for. The book described exactly how I was feeling, what I was thinking, and why I felt so abnormal.

Many of us who have problems with addiction have trauma from the past. We have things we need to deal with. Things we have either gone through or trauma as a result of addiction. For me, being a young woman who got blackout drunk on a regular basis, I ended up in some dangerous situations. Most of the women I know in recovery have significant trauma as a result of the alcoholism. Grief, loss, trauma, even the ability to deal with stress can all be negatively impacted by addiction. These are the things we need to address. Therapy and Eye Movement Desensitization Reprocessing (EMDR) have been very helpful tools (see Resources for more information).

### From surviving to thriving: Tell me a bit about your life today.

When I saw that question, I was like, "Ooh, good question!" I went straight to the dictionary and looked up what "thrive" meant. In reading the definition the word that resonated with me the most was "growth." To thrive we must be growing.

By the end of my drinking days, my world had shrunk significantly. I was completely focused on myself, full of fear and resentment. Life felt very small. In recovery, and especially after hiking the PCT, it became apparent that the world was, in fact, big, bright, and full of possibility. The feeling of realizing I could grow again was powerful.

I felt like a plant that's been stuck in a pot which was way too small for it. You know how it is, the roots get all bound up. Jammed. They can't move. Can't expand. Can't grow. That's exactly how I felt before I stopped drinking. I was lost. Locked into one way of thinking. One way of seeing the world. Stuck in the belief that nothing was ever going to change. All that has shifted—drastically.

Now I feel like I'm rooted deep in the wild earth with unlimited room to grow. My spiritual cup is full. Overflowing. With extra to share.

For me, thriving includes an openness to change. An openness to grow. An openness to doing things differently. An openness to seeing things from a different perspective.

Now, I can see the expansiveness of things. The world, life, the planet, the possibilities. When you are deep in addiction it can feel like you are looking at the sky through a straw. Then, one day, someone comes along and takes the straw away and it's like, wow! Look at the huge sky. It's a wildly different perspective.

Looking back to the backpacking trips in my 20s, I would head out with a platypus full of scotch and tell myself, "I can only walk until this is empty." Today, I can walk anywhere I want. Literally anywhere. There are no limits. I feel like the world is huge. Limitless. That is the feeling I felt when I crested over that mountain pass. Complete freedom. To thrive is to be free.

### If you had one piece of sage advice to offer, what would it be?

In hindsight, I think the worst advice was the advice I gave myself. My mind served me a steady stream of thoughts about my drinking like, "You can control this" and "It's okay, you'll just have to try harder next time" and the classic, "Next time will be different." Of course, it was all B.S. I had been trying to control this disease since I was 12 years old.

From that first day until now, a huge part of my recovery has been learning how to NOT listen to the warped thinking of the addicted brain. I try to stay in the present. I focus on today and try not to get too ahead of myself. To give you an example, about how far my brain was in the future (I laugh now when I think about it). I remember one thought swirling around in my head, telling me that "I couldn't get sober, because I'll have to drink champagne at my wedding..." What's even funnier? At the time, I didn't even have a boyfriend! Yet I could not get that narrow story about some imaginary future event out of my head. So incredibly limiting.

Now, when I catch myself in future thinking, I have learned how to bring my thoughts back to the present. Today I hear a different voice. It reminds me to focus on "What's here. Today. Between now and bedtime." Yes, absolutely, I do my best to live my life like this. Yes, sometimes it's hard. The world is hard. And the future is certainly too elusive to imagine. When I find my mind racing forward, my favorite question for myself is always, "What can I do today?"

Another thing I would say is, "There is hope." I remember my very first AA meeting. A woman was sharing her story. As her eyes connected with mine, she said so sincerely, "You can have a good life." I still get emotional when I think about that moment. At that point in my life, I was in the deepest despair

I had ever felt. I literally didn't think I was going to make it through the next five minutes.

In an instant I felt a glimmer of hope. This kind, brave stranger looked me right in the eyes and gave me hope. I want to offer a ray of hope to someone in despair. I want people to know that, on the other side of addiction, a magical life is waiting for you. Your dreams can come true. Sober, anything is possible...

### Is there anything else you want to add that we didn't cover?

I am living proof. Literally, my biggest dream—hiking the PCT—came true. I never thought I would be able to do that. Yet, three years after getting sober, I was living my dream. If I can do it, you can do it.

In sharing my story, I hope to encourage other people to get the help they need. You don't have to struggle. You pick up the phone. You go online. You take a *Do you Have a Problem with Alcohol* quiz. I passed mine with flying colors. I went to a meeting. Remember, when I went to that AA meeting, I didn't go expecting to quit drinking. I went because I desperately needed help.

Connecting with the AA community saved my life. However, I also want people to know that AA is only one of many ways people can get help. Friends, family, doctors, emergency rooms, Google. The *how* doesn't matter. What matters is that you *do* reach out for help. Do it today!

———

# DIERDRE WOLOWNICK

Rock climber (oldest woman to climb El Capitan)—healing after decades
of enduring a painful, disconnected marriage—rebuilding her life
at 70 through climbing, journaling, and building community

> *"Our minds have a way of zeroing in on the
> dark spots. When we experience nature, on a
> grand scale, in all her glory, she has a way of
> readjusting our viewpoint. Nature has a way of
> putting life back into perspective."*
>
> – Dierdre Wolownick

DIERDRE CAUGHT MY EYE on the cover of an outdoor
magazine. There she was dangling (I am sure that is
not the correct term...) off the side of a massive,
granite rock face, her bright red jacket and the
headline "Setting Records at 50, 60 and Beyond"
with the subheading "Feat: Oldest Woman to Climb
El Capitan, at age 66. If you read the first book in
this series *Never Too Late: Inspiration, Motivation,
and Sage Advice from 7 Later-in-Life Athletes*, you
know that I am a huge fan of real people who
continue to do amazing things regardless of age.

As I read through the article, I learned that
Dierdre, also a writer, had recently published a book
*The Sharp End of Life: A Mother's Story*. I picked up
the book and devoured it. Fascinated by her life

story and knowing she would be perfect for this project, I promptly reached out, introduced myself, and asked for an interview. To my surprise (a part of me always feels surprised when someone says 'Yes'), Dierdre agreed.

Dierdre was born in New York City after World War II. She was raised in an "old world" Polish family with traditional views; children were to be 'seen and not heard' and girls were to serve. By five years old, Dierdre had become her mother's helper; along with that role came the weight of responsibility.

Dierdre's story is one of determination, survival, and triumph. The crux of this conversation highlights the complex layers found in family dynamics, the joys and challenges of intimate relationships, healing through nature, and discovering true joy later-in-life.

I often tell people I work with that "As humans, being in a relationship is one of the hardest things we will ever do…" Dierdre's story validates this truth. I hope the strength, tenacity, and sheer determination of this remarkable woman shines through. With humility and heartfelt gratitude—thank you, Dierdre…

## Dierdre W

*Tell me a bit about you and your background.*

I grew up in New York City (NYC) in the 1950s. It was a fascinating place to grow up. People are often surprised by the amount of nature NYC has to offer—expansive green parks and outdoor spaces. In fact, I think NYC has more green parks than any other city in the country.

I was born into a traditional old-world Polish family. The best way to describe my family growing up was—distant. Emotionally disconnected. In my family, children, especially females, served others. You've heard the classic expression, "children should be seen and not heard?" That was my family's ethos. Personal opinions, wants, desires were dismissed.

My mother survived polio and was very sick. As a result, she had many disabilities. Walking, especially on uneven surfaces, was difficult. Running was out of the question. In general, ordinary balance and movement—which many of us take for granted—was challenging for my mother. By the time I turned five, I had become my mother's helper—basically her surrogate arms and legs. In my family, age was not a consideration. I was a capable female. The caretaking. The fetching. The carrying. It all fell to me. Early in life, I learned how to follow the rules and keep the peace.

Consequently, we didn't do much outdoors as a family. As a child, if I did get out into the woods, go hiking, or go picnicking, it would be with friends or with a friend's family. Sometimes at my grandparents' house we would head outside.

My grandparents lived in Pennsylvania, about a four-hour drive from us. Of course, there were no interstates back then... I remember going there for family events. Holidays and things like that. Our trips to Pennsylvania brought more opportunities to get outside and experience nature.

I also had family who lived in the mountains, north of the city, up in the Catskills. I have fond memories of summers playing with my cousins. There, life felt different. Less heavy. Free. There I was exposed to a lot of nature. Forests. Mountains. Wildlife. I loved it! I remember looking forward to being outdoors, hiking, and exploring.

I have always been an observer. In high school, I had friends who lived on Staten Island. They would take the ferryboat to school every day. I thought that was a grand adventure... As I got older, I could venture out by myself a bit more. I was fascinated by life, by the city, the people, the diversity—by all the details. Over time, I grew to love music, art, and languages. However, people, relationships, and connections seemed elusive—out of my reach.

Fast forward to my mid-20s and a move to southern California. I was finished with college and working as a teacher. The relocation was partly inspired by a family who lived on our block for a brief time. I remember being about five years old when they moved in. The father was a professor. He traveled. The mother, home more, was active, warm, and engaging. They had five children—all blonde! This family was nothing like I had ever experienced.

They were free spirits, exuding freedom and joy. Over time, my dreams about California—palm trees, UCLA, eternal sunshine—became my lifeline. Much to my parents' displeasure.

By this time, I had met Charlie while on vacation. Although physically we had to go our separate ways—Charlie also lived in California—we continued to fuel our romance, long distance with cards, letters, and phone calls. Things fell into place quickly. I secured a teaching job, sold my belongings, packed up the essentials, and moved across the country.

The job came with lodging—and a fast friend—a fellow teacher who shared the villa. The villa, nestled in the middle of a park at the foot of the San Gabriel Mountains, offered direct access to an outdoor wonderland of the likes I had never seen. The trees! Olive trees, orange trees, lemon trees. Avocados growing everywhere. The park was lined with carob trees—their rich, chocolatey scent a constant companion.

As Charlie and I grew closer, we spent the weekends together traveling and exploring. I was in heaven. That first year in California with Charlie was idyllic.

*Diving into the tough topic, tell me a bit about your personal journey/experience.*

The marriage part of my life is an interesting story. Charlie and I decided to get married. The celebration was a whirlwind. Frankly, we would have been happy eloping. Our wedding fulfilled my mother's dreams. The Polish food. The flowers. All the people. Somewhere deep inside, I knew this milestone represented the end of a chapter and the beginning of a new one.

After the wedding, on our way to the airport to catch a plane to our honeymoon destination, I wept a sea of tears. I felt awash with a deep sadness. Grief, loss, and longing. Grief for the closeness I never experienced. Loss for the years of unexpressed emotion. Longing for the warmth of a loving embrace. Charlie held me—silently—as I cried.

My husband was obsessed. He had monomania (an excessive obsession which focuses on one thing). His obsession was mountains. To Charlie, mountains were the only thing that mattered, the only place he wanted to go. Mountains were his everything.

Accordingly, we would go to the mountains—a lot. Yosemite, Lake Tahoe, other places up in the Sierra Nevada. That's what we did while we were dating. That's what we did when the children were small. You may be thinking, "That sounds lovely; what's the problem?" The problem was that it was to the exclusion of *everything* else. Charlie was literally consumed with mountains.

Of course, while we were dating, I had no clue Charlie had an actual disorder. Due to my childhood, I was not well versed in emotions, communication, or consideration about my wants and desires. Plus, in the early days, I thought all this adventuring was wonderful. We would pack up the tent and head off for the weekend away in the great outdoors. Nature and the wonder of it all... Plus, Charlie had a deep knowledge of dry rivers, Indian paintbrush, rain shadows. I was keen to learn.

One night, I remember sleeping on a tarp under a magnificent dome of countless bright stars with the eerie call of coyotes way off in the distance. As we snuggled, I felt warm, protected, safe.

On one of our excursions, through the Sierra Nevada, I saw, for the first time, the majestic eastern wall of the mountains. Those massive slabs of grey granite, rising thousands of feet in the air, spreading out for hundreds of miles as we drove along. That day the skies were crystal clear, I could see the tip of the highest point in California—Mount Whitney. I dreamt about what it would be like to summit Mount Whitney: to stand on the top of the world.

Travel became our life. We talked about our next trip, excursion, or adventure constantly. As soon as we were home from one, Charlie would be ready—planning for the next trip. I was happy and in love.

As the marriage progressed things got worse. A lot worse. Not all at once. It was a slow demise.

Inappropriate remarks. Nasty tones. Disrespect. That sort of thing became common.

Next on the agenda was a move to Japan for teaching positions at a nationally recognized university. Because we had traveled so much, I assumed we knew what to expect. I thought I could handle it. You know, the adjustment. The transition. From the first few hours in Japan, Charlie was unhappy. He hated *a lot* of things. The rain. The rules. The politics. The traffic. Even the language became problematic. In an effort to manage we took opportunities to travel outside the city. We explored the beaches, the castles, the cherry blossoms, and— of course—the mountains. That seemed to help lift Charlie's spirits a bit.

Charlie did not want children. I had dreamt of a large family. Somehow, we found some middle ground. While we were in Japan, our first child was born. A beautiful baby girl.

First-time motherhood, in a foreign land, partnered with a human who was becoming progressively more difficult and disconnected was challenging. Charlie began traveling by himself more regularly. Once again, arriving home from one trip, hanging his hat, and immediately talking, thinking, and planning the next one. The cracks in our relationship became chasms. The isolation, the loneliness, and—at times—the despair became overwhelming.

Three years later, and pregnant with baby number two, we arrived back in the United States. I was so confused. The complete lack of interest. The silence interspersed with outbursts. I began to realize that I was in this relationship—raising children—alone.

Quickly, I became responsible for everything. The chores. The discipline. The holidays. Keeping the peace. Survival. You name it, I did it. This non-marriage made no sense to me...

Money became an issue too. Charlie worked, yet there was no money. There were no discussions and no explanations about money. There was simply, "no money." Our life was in chaos.

In response, I worked. I taught part-time, wrote articles, anything to make ends meet. With the demands of parenting, the jobs, and the house I didn't have time to think, reflect or, frankly, consider what might be wrong with Charlie. With active children in busy phases of their lives— coupled with the hectic pace of my days—the decades rolled quietly along.

On a good day I could convince myself that "life wasn't so bad." We had all the stuff. A home. Opportunities for travel. Involved grandparents. Charlie didn't drink. He didn't gamble. He didn't hit me. He connected with the kids—if the focus was on travel. As long as Charlie could avoid any adult-related tasks like visiting with family, talking to teachers, taking a child to the doctor, he could function. To the outside world Charlie was "quiet, odd." Behind closed doors, Charlie was completely dysfunctional. I was exhausted and overwhelmed.

People assumed we were a typical married couple. So, they treated us like a couple. What they didn't see, behind closed doors, was the complete lack of connection between us. I had no companionship at home—ever. Charlie saw no one. He had no friends. He allowed no friends. No contact with humans. Moreover, there was no opportunity to go out and make friends. I was basically the only adult in the house of four people. The kids were growing up, becoming more adult-like. However, Charlie remained stuck like a defiant child.

In time, my anger swelled, bubbling furiously under the surface. I grew to hate the excursions. Hate the mountains. Hate nature. What once provided solace became filled with frustration, resentment, and angst. Over time, it became evident that nature wasn't the enemy. It was Charlie.

On top of the challenges within the relationship, I went through a span of six years or so where there was nothing but disaster after disaster—inside and outside the family. One of the pivotal events was the deaths of my parents. This left me a house to take care of and an estate to wind down—in another state.

The children were getting older. Of course, they were seeing and understanding more and gaining independence, fast. All the usual things—driving, dating, and thinking about colleges. They were blooming into healthy, strong, capable young adults. By this point, my communication with Charlie had disintegrated to nothing more than the occasional email. I filed for divorce. It was time...

About a month after the divorce was official, I received a phone call: "Mrs. Honnold?" "Yes!" I replied. "Your husband is dead." Charlie had suffered a massive heart attack. In that moment I couldn't breathe. Time stood still. I froze. Although we were divorced, neither of us had time to rewrite wills or express final wishes. Heck, I still had all his belongings.

There was no funeral. No wake. No celebration of life. Alone, I picked up Charlie's ashes. A tiny box— so light and unassuming. Charlie's ashes sat briefly by the fireplace. A fitting gesture: Charlie loved making fires, a skill he prided himself on.

At this point, I was 53, basically widowed, and still alone. This wasn't the life I had imagined. Yet here I was...

After Charlie died, I began connecting with nature again. In fact, that's how I started to come back from this whole morass of disasters. The deaths, the houses to care for, the estates to tie up, the decades of non-stop battering.

Coming full circle, I began hiking again, back out in the Sierra Nevada and the foothills east of

Sacramento. Connecting with nature began to kindle a healing process. Through nature I began to understand what happened, what I dealt with every day. I had turned so much of it off. My thoughts. My feelings. My needs. I couldn't allow myself to process; it was all just too much. Furthermore, because of the marriage, I had no friends, no community, no support. Nature became my companion. My lifeline.

*Please share a little about the role of nature in your healing process.*

When I think about it, nature has always been there. I've always taken great solace in the natural world. Even as a little kid. Walking. Hiking. Just being outside. My mother grew up in a town in Pennsylvania, Hazleton. It was established in 1857 and is located at the foothills of the Pocono Mountains. As I mentioned, we would visit, going back to see her parents, my grandparents, fairly regularly.

When they built Hazleton, they moved a lot of massive, house-sized boulders to the edge of town. Imagine formations of rocks so big they overshadowed the surrounding trees and houses. These giant structures were dumped into the surrounding fields and ravines. This area, known as Mile Rocks, was a wonderful natural playground.

As a child, I remember the grown-ups gathering. All the adults would hang out and talk about who knows what. There were always squabbles. Battles over money, relationships, and seemingly endless family conflict. These conversations bothered me. I recall feeling tense, nervous, and anxious.

To cope, I would go down to the Mile Rocks with the other kids to play, explore, and climb. My first climbing experiences were out on the Mile Rocks. Pretty soon, out in nature, much of the tension would fade away. Everything was good for a moment or two. I felt better. Being outdoors helped soothe the anxiety. Nature has been a consistent backdrop in my life.

I gradually began returning to life. To nature. I started with walking the dog. I had a huge wolf-sized dog. I would take her out, late at night—after my day job and all the estate work. Walking turned into running a little.

Of course, dogs being dogs, she stopped a lot! So, I started leaving the dog at home. In time, I began connecting with a community of like-minded people. I made friends. However, running continued to be a solo endeavor. I had a ridiculous schedule with little spare time. When I did get to run it was often 11 o'clock at night. Nonetheless, I enjoyed running, being outside and this newfound sense of freedom.

Everybody says, "Oh, find a running a partner; an accountability buddy." That wasn't part of my experience. I had my journal. I had my kids. I also had Sacramento with the beautiful foothills, and woods, and running trails. So, it began—rebuilding my life—little by little.

Then climbing entered my life...

About nine years ago, my son (Alex Honnold – rock climber and adventurer) took me to the climbing gym. I was curious. Alex would come home and tell me all about his adventures; I had no clue what he was talking about. From time to time his friends would come over, hang out and talk, using all sorts of different terms and phrases. It felt like a whole new language. I don't like feeling disconnected from what's going on around me. So, I decided to learn about it. Find out what he was talking about. How they do what they do and see if my imagination was correct.

Back then I was a non-climber with no clue about what goes on out there when people go climbing. I had no idea... At that point, I had never even seen climbing in real life. The gear. The terms. The process. It was all new to me and I was keen to learn. So, Alex took me to the gym. He taught me the names of things. How to put on a harness (it's hard to put those things on!) and all about tying in (also known as how to attach the rope to the harness).

We had intended to spend a few hours at the climbing gym. The goal was to learn the bare bones, climb half a wall, and then head home. That's not what happened.

What did happen? Well, it turned out that I climbed 12 walls—all the way up to the top. I wasn't at all worried about looking down—which I had expected. As a kid, growing up in New York with all those huge skyscrapers, I remember looking over the edge or down from a window and feeling my stomach roil. I just assumed I was afraid of heights. As an aside, I often hear people say, "Oh, I could never climb that, I'm afraid of heights." I learned that it's not so much a fear of heights; rather, it's the fear of falling from the height that gets people. When you're on a rope and you know you can't fall from that height—little by little—that fear goes away.

After Alex left, I had to seriously consider this climbing pursuit. I was alone. I didn't know anything or anybody. I was lumpy and overweight. I figured this whole climbing thing was probably not for me.

However, climbing kept calling to me. So, one day, I packed the clothes I needed for the gym and headed there directly after work. I knew that if I went home first, I would waver. I arrived at the gym and started climbing. I loved it! Of course, with climbing came community. Friends. That was 13 years ago.

For the first few months I climbed at the gym with friends. We would meet after work, hang out, climb for the evening, then head back home. It wasn't long before people were inviting me to go along on some of their favorite local outdoor climbs. Well, not exactly local, maybe 60 to 70 miles away in the foothills of the Sierra Nevada. Of course, I jumped at the chance.

I was terrible. I couldn't do anything right. Climbing outdoors is a totally different experience. I felt terrified and frustrated all at the same time. I was a bust! I couldn't get more than eight to ten feet off the ground. I just didn't know what I was doing. My friends were kind and supportive; throughout the climb they offered all sorts of advice, to do this or do that…

It didn't matter that I was terrible, it was fun anyway. I so wanted to figure this climbing thing out. This thing that all these people were doing with such ease. So, I kept going out with them. I kept learning. Kept trying.

One thing about climbing, that makes it a very healing activity, is that it is completely absorbing. You literally cannot think about anything else while you are climbing. You have to laser focus on where your left hand is going. Where your right hand is going. Where your feet are going. What's the angle? Where's the rope going? Where will I hit if I do fall? There's so much to think about when you're climbing. There's no room for thoughts about your job, your marriage, your kids, or anything else.

Climbing out in nature puts you in the zone. It takes you out—far away—from everything else. You are totally focused. In the moment. With the rock. With the rope. That is a wonderfully liberating feeling. So freeing. You are completely unhampered. The worries of life just melt away.

The cool thing about climbing is that each and every time you get out there and climb, you feel this sense of freedom. If you don't fully focus, you won't get up the wall; it's just not possible. For me, that was a huge draw. I had no other release. No other solace. That sense of freedom kept me coming back over and over again. Even the piano and my love for playing doesn't compare to what I feel when I climb. With the piano, I am inside. I am sitting comfortably. I can still think about all the stuff down the hall, the chores, my to-do list.

With climbing, you are outside, moving, and often uncomfortable. It's a totally different experience. When I am out in nature climbing, all the nonsense in my mind melts away. It's amazing. All the pain from the past. All the worries about the future. All swept from my mind—in a flash. It is truly amazing!

Of course, there were many times when I was terrified. I just dealt with it. I think because I was alone for so many years, I knew how to talk myself through things and I learned to just deal...

I remember the first time my climbing buddies took me outdoors. We went on a multi-pitch climb. A multi-pitch takes two people on the rope. One at each end. One climber takes the gear up the wall on their harness. When they have the opportunity, he or she anchors in a piece of gear, making it absolutely secure. Then they attach the rope. This means that if someone falls, they dangle out on that piece of gear, while the person on the ground holds the rope tightly. As a result, they will only fall a few feet. The first climber takes all the risks. If that person doesn't know what they're doing, if they place the gear incorrectly, or make a mistake—the gear will pull out and they will fall. They must know what they are doing. They must do it well. And, they must have complete faith in their equipment. It works like this: the first person heads up, then the second person comes up behind them to a ledge or a pair of bolts where they are hanging. Then they go up again. And again. This technique allows climbers to reach staggering heights.

The first time they took me on a multi-pitch climb I had been climbing for less than a year. I was totally out of my element. There were five or six of us climbing that day. I remember hanging back. Observing. I watched them closely. I did what they told me to do. I made it to the first ledge and I'm thinking, "Okay, first ledge, now I just have to go back down." Not on a multi-pitch, there is no going back down. I got to the ledge, pulled myself up, and sat down. The ledge, of course, faces outward into nothing. You are so high you can see for miles and miles. So high, it's as if you can reach up and pluck a soft, white puffy cloud out of an otherwise clear sapphire blue sky.

I remember glancing down quickly. My mind registered the matchbox-sized buildings and ant-sized people wandering the trails. Then I looked up, and my mind worked hard to make sense of the huge granite wall towering above me. I was absolutely terrified. Paralyzed with fear. I literally froze, I couldn't move.

My compadres kept assuring me, "Here, Dierdre, hold this..." or "Here, Dierdre, tie this on..." "I can't," were the only words I could utter. I was paralyzed with fear. They understood. They left me alone. I just dealt... I tied myself in. Clipped in at several different places. Other climbers had made anchors up there; I think I took advantage of every single one.

I sat there and confronted the fear. I talked myself through it to the point of acceptance, "Okay, I'm here. This is what it is... I am with friends. I'm fine. Breathe." I understood that this feeling was simply fear. I am clipped in four times. I have friends up here with me, nothing bad is going to happen. In reality, I am not in any danger. The fear subsided a little. Developing the skill of talking myself through tough things has been invaluable.

On reflection, I've done an extraordinary amount of talking to myself over the last four or five years.

Particularly as I dangled on the edge of El Capitan, which is 3000 feet tall—that required a lot of internal dialogue.

Sometimes, I wonder if it's a bit different for me because I'm a mom. As a parent my main job for two decades or so was to protect my children from the dangers of the world and, at the same time, keep myself safe so I could be there for them. I was the safety patrol person. I covered the corners of tables. I kept sharp things out of reach. I locked away cleaning supplies. You know, the list is endless... Of course, as a mom, that's your job. Your purpose. Then I go out and do this climbing thing, and somehow I'm supposed to magically forget all that? Yeah, it's not so easy.

I accept that I will never be a super strong "go for it" kind of climber. And that's okay. For me, it's not about being the fastest, the strongest, or the bravest. It's about slowing down, healing and enjoying the moment. Through climbing and being outdoors in this way, I have learned to relax, build relationships, and—maybe for the first time in my life—enjoy people. I feel free to be myself. I have rediscovered a sense of peace and the sense of connection with nature I felt so strongly as a child. In many ways, it's like I have come full circle...

*Is there an experience in nature that stands out in your mind as particularly powerful?*

There have been so many... Each one, has been helpful in its own way. Helpful is a very pale word— but that's what I mean. Each experience has helped my healing process. And, like I said previously, I am still healing. You don't get over things like this in a year. Poof and it's all just gone! It shapes who you are... It shapes your future experiences as well.

As a climber I get to go to the most outrageously beautiful, impressive places that no one else can see. The only way to see these things is to climb up there. That's one thing I have always appreciated about climbing is that you get to experience the world from an incredibly, unique perspective. The view from the top of the El Cap is mind-blowing. Three thousand feet above the valley floor, the summit opens to a seemingly endless panoramic view out over Yosemite Valley and its other famed peaks. It's the most awe-inspiring, humbling experience. It makes me appreciate how small we humans are— how little we matter—in the whole scope of this limitless universe.

Experiences like this—in nature—are key to putting things into perspective. I have found that to be true over and over again. Even if it's just an amble through a green park— whatever—it doesn't have to be a grand outdoor experience.

Sometimes I think that the pace of our human lives has gone awry. When all those deaths were happening, piled up on top of my demanding teaching job, the house repairs, and the estate work—the pace was incredible. Way too much for one person. However, when I'd go climbing everything would slow down. My life, my body, my mind would harmonize again.

When I go up high and look out that snaps everything back into perspective. Nature does that. For me, this has been both powerful and healing. Seeing the full picture is so hard when we are deep in suffering. Whether it's grief or loss or trying to rebuild your life—it's easy to lose perspective when we feel overwhelmed. Our minds have a way of zeroing in on the dark spots. When we experience nature, on a grand scale, in all her glory, she has a way of readjusting our viewpoint. Nature has a way of putting life back into perspective. Nature is calming. She has a pace. A rhythm. For me, that comes through climbing those big walls. For you it may be something different: a walk, a hike, or sitting by a campfire...

*What would you tell people who are currently experiencing what you went through?*

Something basic, which has been very helpful, is journaling. It has been a cornerstone of my healing process. I can't stress that enough. That's how I survived my marriage. I didn't have anybody to talk to. No support system locally. All my friends were either back on the East Coast or overseas. Any family I had was disengaged. I was alone with these horrible things going on. If I hadn't had my journal, I don't know how I would have coped. For me journaling was, and is, immensely helpful.

Next is nature! Get out in nature. Go for a walk. It doesn't have to be some massive hike in the deep woods. Take a walk around the block. Notice things, natural things. The sights. The sounds. The smells. Other people's gardens, window boxes, the trees, the birds. If you can connect with a few of the simple things in your neighborhood, it may be enough to take you away from some of the pain for a moment or two.

Get moving. Walking, running, bike riding, roller skating—it doesn't matter—just get out there. Get that body moving. Breathe. Feel the sun. Look up at the vast sky. Being out in nature, whatever form that takes, can, again, for a moment, push the pause button on the suffering. Space opens up—mentally, physically, emotionally—maybe it's enough to let in a glimmer of a fresh perspective. Hope. Courage. Healing.

When your life is falling apart, when you are suffering, this is so important. Again, it's so easy to zero in on what's wrong, what you can't do, what you haven't got. It's that black and white, all-or-nothing thinking. This mentality can make it seem like this is all there is in the world. Trust me, it's not... get out into nature and see for yourself. Nature will help remind you that there is a big, wonderful world out there full of options and choices and possibilities.

Another thing I might suggest is to reach out to people. Find community. I realize, because of the circumstances, I put relationships way on the back burner. I didn't have the time, permission, or the opportunity. I would have loved to have been able to reach out to a friend or two. To talk. However, my reality, was basically a single parent, running a home, working more than a full-time job, trying to raise children and keep them safe. I didn't have spare moments. At that time friendships felt so far out of my grasp.

### What other tools have been helpful during your healing process?

As I mentioned previously, my biggest—really the only—tool I used was journaling. Remember, I went for decades without a support system. I didn't go out with friends. No get-togethers. No trusted other to lean on. No one to do things with... My journal became my companion.

I wrote. I wrote prodigiously... My journal was my shrink, my therapist, my friend. Journaling was my biggest tool. Journaling, nature, and talking to myself saved my sanity.

*From surviving to thriving: Tell me a bit about your life today.*

Obviously, thriving means different things to different people. I've always been goal driven. I've accomplished a lot of things. I like setting goals and completing them.

For me, thriving means being healthy so I can pursue these goals. Thriving is all about being able to follow my bliss. Follow what I find important in life and to do that healthfully. I still have a lot of goals...

My life today is nice. Everything has changed. I live alone. I have published two books, my memoir: *The Sharp End of Life* and a French textbook. I wrote those, by myself, at home at my dining room table.

I've been climbing a lot. I am also a runner. Over the past four or five years, I have run a whole bunch of road races. I have an office filled with bibs, and numbers, and finishers' medals. My walks around the block blossomed into running 5Ks, half marathons, and then marathons. My daughter, Stasia, is a runner, an endurance athlete. Her "Go, Mommy!" encouragement was infectious. Running, for me, was about balance and power. It was something I could control.

I ran my first marathon when I was 56 years old. I remember sobbing. The tears streamed down my face for many miles. My father had died around this time. I was surprised by the release of the crippling grief I had been holding. Running also taught me how to dig deep—very deep. I didn't realize it at the time—I was running toward a new life. Learning to believe in myself feels like thriving.

Now I have friends. A community. I like seeing them. We hang out. Have lunch. Climb. I love to write. I enjoy public speaking. I love to travel. I love absorbing foreign languages. Plus, there are so many beautiful rocks all over the world—I want to climb them all. Climbing abroad is a large part of what I want to do for my next decade.

The French Alps. The Dolomites in Northern Italy. Switzerland. Canada. I want to climb in Japan, where there is wonderful limestone climbing. I want to go back to Mexico and its wonderful climbing. I'd also like to try South America. Little by little. Baby steps…

### If you had one piece of sage advice to offer, what would it be?

When our world is falling apart, things are horrible, and we can't see any light at the end of the tunnel. Some people respond by shutting down, internalizing, drawing inward, concentrating on themselves. I see this as an important part of the healing process. You have to focus on you. Some people think this is "selfish." It's not selfish, it's survival!

That's what journaling is about. That's what running is about. That's what getting out in nature is about. All these things will help you navigate through the rough times.

Please, connect with other people. My life didn't really start to change until I connected with other like-minded people. Meeting my climbing crowd—hanging out, exchanging stories, sharing lives, feeling like somebody cares, gets me, and understands—has been huge. Incredibly healing.

Building community can take many forms. You can go and volunteer at a soup kitchen. Consider using your talents and skills. I played piano duets at the senior center for a while. They loved it. For me, it was such a warm, enriching experience. In those moments nothing else existed. Read to school children. Clear trails for your local park. Find something that will get you out of yourself and into that zone so that you can forget those worries—for just a little while. Even an hour or so can help. It's enough to send you back refreshed—ready to deal with it again.

*Is there anything else you want to add that we didn't cover?*

Throughout these trials in our lives, what's important is the depth to which you know yourself. Take some time to learn about who you are. Make sure you understand your values and what's important for you. Without this self-knowledge it's easy to get distracted, flounder, and pulled away from your life's course.

It's the opposite of the "try this" message our media-driven culture bombards us with. Try this food, try that drug, try this lifestyle. What they don't know is who *you* are, what *your* body needs, and what *your* mind requires. There's so much bad advice out there. Moreover, that bad advice is constantly changing. Admittedly, I'm out of touch with the world. I don't watch television. I don't sit around talking about the latest gossip, drama, or scandal. I believe I am better off for it...

Recently, at a friend's house, I happened to catch the ads on a cable news channel. I was standing to leave and noticed every single ad was for a drug. A drug to lose weight. A drug to help you sleep. A drug to wake up. Drugs for your children. Drugs for your pets. I was absolutely appalled. Our natural state does not involve taking manufactured pharmaceuticals. That's not who we are. Yet, these companies are making billions of dollars. It's marketing. That's all it is. Unfortunately, people believe it.

In short, any healing process *has* to start with you and understanding who you are and what you value. Sadly, many people don't take the time to consider these foundational elements.

I, of course, journaled… If you decide journaling might be a helpful part of your process, start with questions like, "What do I want from my life? Why do I want this? What do I cherish? What are my values? Where did these values come from?" These are the kinds of things we should all be thinking about regularly. This is where the healing process begins to unfold.

Finally, know that healing is possible—it takes time, sometimes a lifetime, yet it is possible. Healing takes quiet. It takes time out in nature. In today's world there are so few opportunities to be alone with ourselves. To reflect on our thoughts, our feelings, our hopes and our dreams, to really connect with who we are on a deeper level. Nature is steadfast, and always offers us the gift of solitude that can help us heal.

———

# SALLY ADAMS

A nurse on the front lines during COVID—healing debilitating anxiety—through bike touring, walking, and rediscovering balance through nature

*"...the fact that I could make myself feel like I mattered in the world felt good. That's how powerful being outside and being active has been for me."*

– Sally Adams

SALLY IS A 45-YEAR-OLD self-proclaimed Gen-Xer and a "recovering perfectionist" who spent much of her life in "catch-up mode." Sally grew up in Minnesota, a state within the United States which borders Canada and Lake Superior. It's famous for its water, with more than 10,000 lakes dotted throughout the state. Minnesota is also home to many other natural wonders. For instance, Niagara Cave, formed by water erosion over millions and millions of years. Today, visitors can explore a labyrinth of underground passages and witness many stalagmites and stalactites exquisitely sculpted by the hand of Mother Nature.

Sally's story struck me because it's a narrative I think we can all relate to. Nothing wild. Nothing over the top. No deep childhood wounds. Simply a woman working hard to do all the right things in life.

With a relatively happy childhood, Sally did well in school. She got good grades and had a strong social network. After high school, Sally decided to go to nursing school which meant less time, more pressure, and even higher expectations. The demands of nursing school where soon traded for the break-neck pace of life—and the reality of working in a busy emergency department. Then COVID hit, bringing with it unprecedented levels of stress, exhaustion, and anxiety.

Sadly, in the midst of the pandemic, Sally's mother passed away—in the same emergency department—adding another layer of trauma and loss to Sally's world. Pushed to her limits with little time for rest, relaxation, or self-care—overcome with debilitating anxiety—Sally's mind and body crashed. At one point, Sally was so deeply entrenched in anxiety and disconnected from everything around her, that her therapist literally prescribed a daily walk around the block. Which, in the depth of a Minnesota winter, is no trivial feat. Yet, a small part of Sally knew this "walk" was more than just exercise—it was about survival. She bundled up and got out there. For Sally, this was a turning point.

In my experience, having anxiety is often pathologized, dismissed, or minimized... This conversation normalizes anxiety, helping us see how it can build over time, and that no one is immune—while at the same time, offering us some insight, tools, and coping strategies. I hope, through Sally's journey, you too will connect with the power—and importance—of movement, nature, kindness, grace, and self-compassion. Thank you, Sally, for sharing your courageous story!

## Sally A

*Tell me a bit about you and your background.*

I am a Gen-Xer—a child of the 80s. I have lived my whole life in Minnesota. I identify as a Minnesotan. I've had the joy of growing up in a state with all four seasons. Even though two of the seasons—spring and fall—while gorgeous, are very short. The climate lends itself to spending a ton of time outside. Whether it be the dead of winter or mid-summer, we spend time outdoors.

My family didn't 'do' a lot of outdoorsy things. However, growing up, the message was "go outside, find your friends, and play." Minnesota is known as the "Land of Ten Thousand Lakes." Consequently, spending time on the water is a big deal. I was fortunate that my grandparents lived on a lake in central Minnesota. As kids, we would spend the summers out on the water, playing from dawn to dusk—burning our skin tomato red—loving every moment of it.

To this day, I remember being out on the dock hearing the sound of the water, feeling the breeze coming off the lake, spending time with friends and family, and connecting with a deep sense of joy and relaxation. I absolutely loved it! My family was lower-middle class. As a kid, a part of me knew having access to my grandparents' lake home was a privilege—something really special.

During the summers, we would be by the water or camping at the local state parks. In the winter it was time for cross-country skiing. I remember my dad spending his summers scouring garage sales and local goodwill stores for the gear we needed for the winter ski season.

I guess it wasn't so much that my family was into the outdoors. In fact, the memories from our camping trips include my parents bickering as they worked to put up the tent. Although our camping vacations seemed stressful for the adults, for us kids it was so much fun. I think spending so much time outside was more a reflection of our circumstances. We didn't have much money to do other things; the outdoors and the natural world was our entertainment. I also think it was the era. After school, we were left to our own devices. We were latchkey kids, often fending for ourselves or hanging out with friends. Sometimes our parents were home, and busy; the message was, "Go outside and play."

As I got older—into high school—I got involved in athletics. For me, life in high school was all about friends, fitting in, and extra curriculars; spending time outside faded into the background. It was a similar story during my college years. There, my life was focused on going to class, working, getting that degree, and trying to figure out the direction of my life. It was like I was in this cycle of work, school, work, school, work, school. That was the grind. I did it for a lot of years.

Today, I find myself feeling a little bit envious when I see videos online of young people in their late teens or early 20s who have somehow figured out a way to incorporate nature, hiking, traveling, and school into their lives. It's neat to see young people living in a more balanced way.

In fact, I've commented to friends over the years that growing up, I didn't know there was another option, an alternative to the daily grind. When I was in high school, I remember being asked repeatedly, "Where are you going for college?" and, "What are you going to major in?" It wasn't part of our family's DNA to talk about trade schools or gap years or other options. I think part of that comes from my dad's experience. He went into the Marine Corps right out of high school. My dad placed a high value on education. Interestingly, he graduated from college the same year I graduated from high school. We were conditioned—that's just what you do.

As a result, I basically spent a whole decade—from 20 to 30—going to school and working. I am not complaining. It's got me to where I am today. I am grateful for that. However, I was so focused and driven, it didn't occur to me to take some time to stop and smell the roses. So, yes, during those years there was a big gap in my self-care and no time spent outside in nature.

*Diving into the tough topic, tell me a bit about your personal journey/experience.*

Because I spent a decade focusing on getting my education and figuring out where my career was going, my physical and mental wellbeing suffered. I started smoking. I was in nursing school learning about the myriad of health consequences from smoking when I was finally able to quit. I was working two jobs; nights at the hospital, waiting tables during the day—just trying to pay the bills. My food habits were horrible, and the concept, or time, to exercise might as well have been a million miles away.

By the time my early 30s rolled around, life began to balance out a bit. I had been nursing for a couple of years when a co-worker invited me to do a Tough Mudder. The run consisted of navigating 25 obstacles spread over 12 miles. My friend was like, "Girl, we're getting a team together. It's going to be awesome. You have to do it!" Keep in mind, I was not in shape. Yes, occasionally I might do 30 minutes on the elliptical but my whole life was still basically in catch-up mode. I remember thinking to myself, "Why would I want to do that? I'm not a runner. It sounds miserable." Then he shared that this event was dedicated to raising money for a cause that was close to my heart. My thinking quickly changed, "Well heck, if it's going to be a team thing and it's going to raise money for this cause, I'm in!" My next thought was, "Well, I'd better get running."

So, I started running. It was miserable. I hated every second of it. My body seemed to reject every step. One day, I remember hitting the two-mile mark. I was like, "Wow! How did I manage that?" I continued to train for this event and added strength training to my exercise schedule. I trained hard for about six months. Race day finally came; I felt nervous and scared. It was me with four male team members. As the only female on the team, I was afraid of being the weakest link. Unbeknownst to me, I had been overtraining. As a result, I was able to keep up with one of my favorite, incredibly fit co-workers. We crushed it!

So, while it was a super scary experience, in the end I felt so proud of myself. Plus, in the process of training for that event, I learned a lot about my own strength, determination, and my ability to overcome fear. It was life changing. I remember thinking,

"Gosh, I just did all this work, I might as well keep going. I wonder if I could I run ten miles? What about a half-marathon?" So, I set more goals and kept on running.

I was sharing with my significant other recently, that doing this helped me learn that as an adult, I am capable. I spent a lot of time in my youth and young adult years feeling like I had no value. That I wasn't particularly special. That I wasn't particularly interesting. Despite the fact that, from the outside, I had always seemed very independent, very determined, very dedicated. I graduated from college with top honors. I bought my first house when I was 22, blah, blah, blah... However, none of it felt like an accomplishment. I didn't feel worthy—even worthy of my own respect. When I started doing these physical activities, achieving these goals, it was less about the physical aspect, and more about the recognition that I was mentally capable. For the first time, I felt strong, confident, determined, and dedicated. I felt proud of myself. For the first time, I felt like I had value. Because I had spent much of my life feeling like a failure, a disappointment, this was a big deal for me.

As an adult in my 30s, I am for the first time feeling good about myself. Like I am something. Like I'm cool. Trust me, it doesn't mean that I'm not still a totally-flawed human or that I think I am high and mighty, looking down on everyone else. It means

I have self-respect. That I have positive thoughts and feelings about myself—in a healthy way—and that's okay. The fact that I could make myself feel like I mattered in the world felt good. I also realize that I am capable of much more than I ever thought. That's how powerful being outside and being active has been for me.

### Please share a little about the role of nature in your healing process.

After being a nurse for about three years, I decided to take a job in the emergency department (ED). I was excited to be in a new environment. I was looking forward to sinking my teeth into something new. About six months into the new job, I developed horrible, horrible anxiety. I realized I was intellectually fully capable of working in that environment. My skill set and my work ethic were perfect for the ED. However, I was not, in any way, prepared emotionally or mentally for what it would be like to work in that environment. I just had no idea. The mental/emotional strain of the job never came up. I didn't know anyone who was a first responder. My prior experience included caring for heart patients and a stint in labor and delivery. I honestly thought the ED would be an easy transition. Boy, was I wrong!

Over time, the anxiety became debilitating. I woke up every day feeling a sense of overwhelming fear. I couldn't leave the house. I didn't want to see friends. It was intense. I knew something was very wrong. I called my primary care doctor. I told him all about my symptoms. He started me on some medication and suggested I connect with a therapist to develop some behavioral strategies. The medication he prescribed to help with the anxiety was awful. After a week, I felt so groggy. So weird. Through the fog a part of me thought, "I can't do this..." I stopped taking the medication.

Thankfully, by that time I had connected with a therapist. He helped a lot. He helped me understand anxiety, what it is, what was happening in my body, and helped me develop strategies to manage the anxiety. The first thing he did was encourage me to find things that helped my body feel relaxed. Things that took my mind off the intense feelings of fear and panic. So, I started exploring things... For instance, I had never had a massage; that was the first thing I tried. I also began taking walks in the nature center close to where I grew up. Pretty quickly, I started to realize that being out in nature helped me feel a bit better. When I was outside, I felt okay, more relaxed, less afraid. The therapy and re-connecting with nature worked hand-in-hand. The more I used these strategies, the more I noticed I started feeling better.

Do I still struggle with anxiety? Yes. Particularly health anxiety, mostly triggered by the things I saw in the ED. I worked there for 12 years—longer than anyone should ever be in that environment. I figured out ways to cope with the anxiety, manage what I saw, and the things I was exposed to. There were reasons why I stayed there as long as I did. I worked with some amazing people and took a lot of pride in my work.

Overall, I think I have a fairly typical life. I didn't suffer childhood trauma. I didn't lose a parent at a young age. I haven't had cancer. I haven't had any catastrophic events I have had to overcome. Of course, I've had regular life stuff—relationship challenges, family dynamics, work stressors, etc. Yet, here I am, battling debilitating anxiety.

Struggling with anxiety has made me slow down. For the first time in 30 plus years, I have had to learn about myself. Look inside. Figure out what's going on... I spent so much of my time on automatic pilot—driving through life, trying to reach a destination. Staying active and being outside has played a huge role in my recovery. Nature is my pathway to healing.

I work in an acute care hospital; COVID has been extremely challenging. Things are changing every day. It's hard and scary. You just can't get away from it... The fear was everywhere: family, friends, co-workers, social media, news—all talking about COVID. Then I went to work and swam in it all day long—it got really hard. I got to a point where acute depression started to settle in on top of the anxiety. I recognized it. My therapist recognized it. I remember my therapist asking, "Are you having any thoughts of harming yourself?" I wasn't. He recognized I was in a dark place. I couldn't remember the last time I smiled, laughed, or felt joy.

It was clear the depression was situational—the result of being a frontline healthcare worker and everything we endured during the pandemic. I remember my therapist asking, "Okay, what are you doing for yourself? What are you doing right now?" I was like, "Nothing. Absolutely nothing." His response was immediate, "Okay, we're done for today. You're going to go take a walk..." Keep in mind, this was mid-December in Minnesota and 28 degrees outside. A big part of me was saying, "This is going to suck..." The therapist, probably seeing the look on my face, said, "It doesn't matter how far or how long you go. Just do something for yourself." I said, "Okay." I got off the Zoom call (remember, it's 2020 and telehealth sessions). I put on my hat and my scarf and my Sorel boots and my down jacket and I walked down the block and back. It was the most physical activity I'd done outside of work, and it was the most time I'd spent outside in months.

I felt proud of myself. The fresh air made me feel human again. I think it was the sound of nothing that struck me. There was no TV, no phones, no radio. There were no cars on the road. All I could hear was the wind rustling the trees and my feet crunching over the snow-covered ice. I felt the fresh, cold air sting my face. The deeper breaths forced me to reset. To adjust my mindset. My therapist was right: I did need to take care of myself. A short walk around the block was a good start.

Since then, I have developed the mentality that anything counts. Anything you do for yourself matters. Walking down the block and back—counts. Sitting outside on my front step drinking tea for ten minutes or so—that counts. Watching the geese on the pond. Noticing the butterflies bask and play and flitter around. Plus, time I spend doing things that connect me with nature—it all counts. All of it helps me rest my soul so I can go on and be there for others.

During that dark time, I started making the effort to get outside more often. Before long, I was walking all the way around the block. Then I would go a little bit further. Even if it was once or twice a week, I knew it was good for me. It felt good to care about myself again. Inside, I began to feel more peaceful, more beautiful. I began to believe it would be okay. Like I would be okay.

Making that commitment to get outside and walk was a turning point. Once the weather started to get nicer, I started to run a little. Pretty soon, the summer hiking season arrived, and in Minnesota that's always a big deal because it means long days outdoors.

The hiking is amazing in Minnesota. We are gifted with incredibly beautiful places to hike. What's special about hiking compared to taking a walk or going for a run, is that you can remove yourself from humanity. I cherish being in the woods where there's little evidence of other people. All I hear is the sound of water and the whisper of leaves. I remember a particular hike, in the spring that year, when I stopped still in my tracks and noticed a feeling of complete peace. Just me, making my way over the rocks and roots. Noticing the sound of the grouse which, if you haven't experienced, is unbelievable. In these moments, I am aware that my body is physically responding—in a good way. I can feel my brain slow down and begin to relax. Because my life is full of distractions, diversions, and busyness, it is very hard for me to connect with this level of peace and tranquility. Hiking, in particular, helps me unplug.

### Is there an experience in nature that stands out in your mind as particularly powerful?

A couple of years ago, I was in a relationship with somebody who rode a motorcycle. We did a lot of traveling on the bike. We would take these long road trips from Minnesota out West—Colorado, Utah, South Dakota, and Wyoming. I remember experiencing nature in a way that was so therapeutic. All I did was ride along on the back of that bike and watch the world pass by. The beauty I was seeing and the smells I was smelling were awe-inspiring. I particularly remember the lilac bushes in full bloom. I'll never forget that rich, sweet fragrance. It's equally memorable to ride past something dead— phew, awful. I'll remember that too...

Judgement aside, experiencing the natural world from the back of a bike was one of the most powerful, peaceful, and rich sensory experiences I have ever had. During these long trips, nature took on a whole new meaning. I felt the majesty of the mountains and the openness of vast prairies. I rode toward the first rays of sun as it lit up the sky. It all touched me very deeply. I have had similar feelings while hiking the north shore of Lake Superior. Each time I feel this way, I try to remember that it doesn't take a whole lot to start the healing process.

I desperately wanted to feel better. Somehow, I knew nature could help. With time, encouragement, and practice I learned how to be present. To be vulnerable. I learned that I could sit with my best friend and cry. I learned to sit on the shore of Lake Superior and simply soak in the sunset.

In these natural remote places, away from all the artificial assaults on the senses, I found the courage to heal and forgive. To forgive myself. To forgive people who have harmed me. To let go of the anger, the sadness, the pain. Nature showed me how to open a door and welcome in peace, contentment, and harmony. Was it a slow process? Yes. Yet, miraculously, as the moments, the experiences, and the feelings began to meld together, I was able to let some of the old stuff go. I began noticing fresher, lighter, more peaceful energy creeping into my mind and body.

Of course, all of the things that are circling in my life are still there. It's not like they magically disappear. It's just okay to let them go for a while. When I'm deep in the woods or hiking or at the lake, I'll lay on the beach for a while. I'll listen to the movement of the water. I'll notice the light changing in the sky. Soon my mind begins to slow down a little and my body begins to rest. I begin to feel okay again. Yes, my life and all its challenges are still there but—right now—I can give my brain a break from all that. It's such a gift.

We spend so much of our time busy—striving, doing, accomplishing. It's like there is this hidden message that if you are not striving, doing, and accomplishing, then you are "lazy" or "complacent" or "not enough;" at least that's how it felt for me. Now, I realize that contentment is equally important and, in some ways, a lost art. Through all this, I am discovering that there is something liberating about having the ability—in this moment—to accept where I am, what I have, and who I am without judgement.

*What would you tell people who are currently experiencing what you went through?*

My advice? Try anything. For me, since having anxiety and panic attacks, regular old therapy has been a staple in my life, which has been so helpful. As a healthcare professional, I encourage people to find something to help get outside of themselves. Maybe it's a walk at the local park. Maybe it's bowling. Maybe it's time with friends. Whether you think you're capable of it or not—give it a try. Even if you find yourself thinking, "This looks awful," give it a try. If there's a chance it helps you feel better or disconnects you from the minutiae of life—give it a try!

I also encourage people to explore activities that help you feel connected to yourself. Things that help you think more clearly. Activities that allow you to be kinder to yourself. I am an introvert. In my world, it feels good to do nothing for an entire day. I'll watch reruns of old TV shows I love. Often, I won't talk to another soul—that feels great.

Remember, there are people all over the planet that are struggling with something. Everything from big scary stuff—grief, loss, illness—to all sorts of daily challenges—school, jobs, family. This is particularly true, right now. With COVID, there is so much grief, loss, and trauma.

As I reflect, there were times in my healing journey when I felt discouraged, defeated, and completely unsupported—quite alone. I wanted external support but couldn't seem to find it. Because I didn't have supportive parents or a supportive partner—someone validating me—somehow, I felt like what I was doing or trying was wrong or not valid.

Today, my life is different. I am fortunate. I have some amazing people in my circle. Now I can look back and see that a part of me wanted, or needed, other people to be on my journey with me. However, that just wasn't the reality. Somehow, going it alone helped me feel capable, strong. It gave me a lot of pride. Going it alone allowed me not to compare myself to others. The truth is—we are all unique. This is your journey and your healing process. What matters is whether what you are trying is helpful or unhelpful—for you. Is what you're doing working for you? Are you feeling any better? More balanced? More complete? These are important questions to be asking yourself.

Lastly, if you are trying something new, don't be discouraged by someone else's lack of interest. Whether it's a walk around the block, a bike ride, or some quiet time listening to the birds... If what you are doing is meeting your needs, helping you feel a bit better, it's valid.

*What other tools have been helpful during your healing process?*

Obviously, different things resonate with different people. When I started struggling with anxiety I turned to books. For me, reading, mostly self-help books, has been a huge help. Over the years, there have been a couple of books. One in particular that I pull out now and again is called *Rapid Relief from Emotional Distress*. It's an oldie, published in the 1980s. It's marked up all over the place, and the pages are torn and yellowed. It's been a great resource.

I am lucky to have some awesome people in my life. People I trust. People I can be completely transparent with. Developing deeply honest, loving friendships was huge for me. It doesn't matter whether you are in the same phase of life or whether you have different interests, knowing there is at least one person in my corner has been invaluable.

Here's a good example, I have a friend: we met at the hospital, and we're thick as thieves. She was very present when my mom died a few years ago. My mom's death was complicated. She died unexpectedly in the emergency department I work in. Like I said, it was complicated. We had to raise money to cover the funeral and other costs. Then there was the trauma of having to be around the room where she died. My friend was with me all the way. It's funny, because she and I are so different. For instance, she thinks camping is utter nonsense and wants nothing to do with hiking. Yet, despite our differences, we love and support each other completely. I am so grateful for her. It's that sense of knowing you are not alone in your struggles.

*From surviving to thriving: Tell me a bit about your life today.*

My mom and I had a challenging relationship. She was an amazing person with a good heart, yet for various reasons, our relationship was strained. She was 69 when she died. As I mentioned earlier, she died where I worked. Emotionally, that was a huge challenge for me. With the help of a wonderful therapist who specialized in grief, I decided to go back to work—in the same department. There has been a lot of healing around the loss of my mom. That for sure has been a transition from surviving to thriving.

Through this journey we call life, I am learning that there will always be challenges, setbacks, disappointments, and hard decisions we all have to make. And, at times, there will be hurt, loss, and sometimes a lot of pain. I am realizing that I can—and will—survive.

Also, I know that the decisions I make about how I take care of myself are the difference between me surviving or me thriving. Last winter, I was surviving. Literally, trying to get through each day and be okay. That's also how I felt when my mom died. I was focused on trying to get through the next shift at work without going into the room where she died. With time, it's got a little easier.

Now, when I have challenges with my significant other or I am feeling sad about something or anxious or depressed, I try to remember that this is a moment in time and there's a lot to be grateful for. I am fortunate and privileged. I have a healthy body. I have people who love me.

In my mind, the difference between surviving and thriving is fluid. A continuum. It moves back and forth, ebbs and flows. We have phases of thriving intertwined with times when it is all about surviving. Regardless of the phase I am in, I try to stay positive and grateful. Yes, sometimes I fail miserably. Other times, I handle it like a superstar. Sometimes you run a half marathon and sometimes you walk around the block—and that's okay.

Seeing surviving and thriving as a continuum has helped me because they are not "all or nothing" concepts. Over the lifespan, there will be steps forward and there will be steps backward. We are constantly moving through these cycles. When life is good, I try to recognize it and be in a place of gratitude.

I think that's the power of nature. Nature helps me be present—grounded in the moment—regardless of whether I am surviving or thriving. A million years ago, I studied a little about Buddhism. Buddhists see all of life as a constantly changing flow of events. When I can stand back a bit and see the valleys of life as simply a valley and the peaks of life as simply peaks—in that moment I feel like I am thriving.

### If you had one piece of sage advice to offer, what would it be?

If there's one thing I want people to take away from my story, it is *please* be kind to yourself. Often, we are our own worst critics. I am no exception. I wish I had learned to be gentler, kinder, more self-accepting earlier in my life.

Also, remember to focus on the positive things. Admittedly, it is sometimes hard to find them, but they are there. List them out: I am capable. I am kind. I am a loyal friend. I am good at organizing closets—whatever... Speak to yourself, in your internal dialogue, as if you are a cherished child or beloved grandparent. If I had spent as much time seeing myself through my grandmother's eyes versus the relentless critic's eyes, I'd be much better off.

### Is there anything else you want to add that we didn't cover?

I am grateful for the opportunity to share a tiny part of my story. I am a regular everyday person; if my story helps someone else even a tiny bit—that's amazing!

Lastly, remember that our journeys are different. Sometimes life is simple; other times, it's complicated, painful, and messy. Even though our experiences may be very different, collectively, as humans, we are more similar than we are different. We're on this planet—for who knows how long—be kind, move, get out in nature, and know we are all trying to do our best.

———

# WILL SPROUSE "IRON WILL"

Ultra-runner—healing after a devastating motorbike crash and a massive stroke—rebuilding his life through running, nature, and incredible willpower

*"The fact is that running a hundred miles is a lot like life. You will hit low points. You will feel like quitting. If you can learn to push through the low points, your body—and brain—will find a way to overcome the adversity."*

– Will Sprouse

**WOW! WILL SPROUSE** is also known as "Iron Will"— for good reason. I'm speechless. What an incredible story. Will has been through so much. So many highs; so many lows, including a full recovery from a terrible motorbike accident where the doctors assured him that his running days were over. As an ultra-runner, not walking—let alone never running again—was not an option. Will takes us through his experience from being physically broken to crushing those ultra-races again.

As you know, life often tests us… Will's story is the epitome of this sentiment. After winning his first Slam race (a series of four 100-mile races scheduled pretty much back-to-back—yes, you read that right!), things were really taking off for him in the ultra-running world. Then COVID hit, the country was shutting down, and events and races were being cancelled. In the fall of that year, Will had a massive stroke. This time the prognosis was life in a wheelchair...

I am both honored and humbled to share more about this incredible man. Will's story gives us a glimpse of the depth of the power—mental and physical—we, as humans, are capable of. He discusses intuition, determination, and the importance of listening to—and harnessing—our natural wisdom and our innate ability to heal. With much gratitude, here's Will...

### Will S

*Tell me a bit about you and your background.*

My dad was in the military, so I was born in Germany. We lived there for 11 years. I was very sick when I was born. I was on life-support. My parents were told that I probably wouldn't make it through the night. Thankfully the doctors were wrong. I survived and became a "miracle baby."

As a result, I was in the hospital for the first three months of my life. My lungs kept filling up with fluid and I had issues breathing. Plus, I had a heart defect—which I didn't learn about until recently. I actually had it repaired recently (more about that later).

With a dad in the military and growing up in Europe, we had a lot of opportunity to be outdoors. I remember going fishing with my dad. He was also into Volksmarching—a form of non-competitive outdoor walking. I recall our long walks—miles and miles—through the Black Forest in Germany. As kids, my brother and I loved running through the forest. I really enjoyed that.

For the most part, I grew up in large cities like Frankfurt and Stuttgart, Germany. To get to any forest would involve an hour and a half drive—yet that didn't seem to stop us.

When we came back to America we settled in Kansas. Our new home was in more of a small-town environment. I went to high school in Kansas, where I was active, into sports, and in good shape.

When we got back stateside, I did more hunting and fishing with my dad. I wasn't much for hunting, but I enjoyed time outdoors with my father. I was also a Boy Scout—that's where I learned all about the woods and surviving in the wilderness. In my late teens, once I moved out of the house, the hunting and the Boy Scouts ended.

After high school, I went to college. This is when my life changed a lot. I worked and took a full load of courses. I also quit sports and stopped any physical activity.

After college I went into the restaurant business. Specifically, a management position. Leadership roles in this industry are known for long, demanding hours. During the day, although I was around food all the time, I didn't eat. After work, I'd arrive home, generally late at night, starving. I would sit down and eat a full meal—and more—then fall asleep. There was no time for movement, exercise, or anything else really. The bad health habits continued. By the time I was 35 years old, I weighed over 300 pounds.

My dad was a marathon runner. He was good; so good, that he ran for the military. I could never comprehend how he could run so far. Anyway, sadly, my dad got cancer. He fought it hard for 12 years. I was 35 years old when he died.

So, here I was… mid-way through my 30s. Working 24/7, 300-plus pounds, and my father was dead. Furthermore, I had multiple health concerns. My doctor's message was loud and clear, "You won't be around much longer if you don't make some lifestyle changes." I knew they were right. So, to cope with my dad's death and my failing health, I started running.

I committed to running six days a week. At first, I could only manage a couple of steps around the block. I would run, walk, run, walk. Although it felt hopeless at times, I kept at it. By the three-month mark, I was up to three miles a day, six days a week. Then, fairly soon after that, I was running ten miles a day—six days a week! I just kept on going, adding more and more miles.

At the six-month mark, I had lost over half my body weight. I was down to a much healthier 150 pounds. I decided it was time to start running marathons. I wasn't superfast. It was a good day if I could finish in under four hours.

The running bug hit me hard. I ran a couple of marathons a month. Then I progressed to back-to-back marathons on weekends. Up to this point, it was all road running.

Around June 2008, due to the warm weather, heat, and humidity, I started having trouble finding road marathons. I managed to find a race located in the Black Hills of South Dakota called the Mickelson Trail Marathon. It was basically a rail-trail course. This was the first time I switched from pavement (street or road running) to trail running. The terrain wasn't super rough. I remember running that first trail race, going through the Black Hills, the trees, the ponderosa pines, the wildlife, the rolling hills—it was stunning. I was hooked!

July came. And another trail race, 50 miles. This time in Wisconsin in the Devils Lake area. The 350-plus acre lake is protected by gentle bluffs that rise along the shoreline. I remember the water that day, pristine, crystal clear, and shimmering blue. These were real trails—trees, rocks, roots—and challenging. This was my first ultra. It was horrible.

*Diving into the tough topic, tell me a bit about your personal journey/experience.*

In 2010, I just finished a 50-miler in Indiana. It was one of the Dances with Dirt—the Gnaw Bone Series. Man, those hills were brutal. The following weekend I was riding my motorcycle to work when, out of nowhere, a big dog, hidden by the weeds, jumped out right in front of my motorbike. I hit him square on at 60 miles per hour. It was bad. I flew over the handlebars and careened down the road.

I landed down on the asphalt, unable to breathe, gasping for air as my lungs were quickly filling up with blood. Emergency services arrived on the scene. It was chaos. Basically, from the shoulders down, my body was crushed. I was flown by helicopter to a local trauma center. I had all kinds of internal bleeding. I fractured 46 bones. Everything from my shoulders down to my hips was crushed, including my pelvis.

Thankfully, I didn't have any damage to my head—everything from my shoulders up and my legs were fine. I did break my big toe; I guess it got caught on the bike as I was being thrown into the air. Twenty-three of my ribs were completely shattered, splintering off into my insides. That's where all the internal bleeding was coming from.

I survived, of course... I was basically told to find another hobby. How did the doctor word it? Oh, yes, "Because you'll probably never run again."

Somehow, in all the chaos they missed the broken pelvis. That injury wasn't discovered until later. The doctors wanted to re-break it and reset it. I said, "No." As a result, my left side is a little shorter than my right side—I've learned to cope with it.

Even though I was healing, I kept having recurring bleeding in my thoracic area. Shards from the shattered ribs would punch through some of my good ribs. I had to get blood drained on a regular basis. Oh, and my back was broken in ten places.

I guess I did a somersault through the air. My shoulder took the brunt of the fall, and then I flipped onto my back as my body hit the pavement. I was in recovery for about three months. That was another challenge. I was doped up on so much morphine and oxycontin. The whole thing was a blur. I slept all the time. I felt completely worthless. I just couldn't do it anymore.

I was determined to get back to running.

I got tired of feeling disconnected and sleeping all the time. They had me so doped up, I don't recall much of that period. Three months of my life, evaporated, in a hazy fog. So, I decided to take myself off all the drugs. I told the doctors, "I'd rather be conscious and live with some pain."

When I started weaning off the drugs, I began to feel my body again. It was amazing. I started noticing pain in places that had not been identified as problematic. With a clearer head, I could listen to my body and communicate with the medical people, "Hey, doc, I have pain here; something's wrong there…" A bone scan was ordered which revealed 46 broken bones instead of the original 27, along with evidence of a broken pelvis, previously missed by the doctors.

Like I said, I'm stubborn. I was getting back to running.

The accident happened in May of 2010, Memorial Day weekend. About nine months after the accident, I was back to running. I signed up for a 50K called the Black Warrior. The course was quite technical: river crossings, rocks, roots, etc. It took me about six hours to finish the race. Slow compared to my pre-accident times, but hey, I finished! I was very happy to be back and running.

Next, I wanted to experiment with a 100-mile race. Later in that same year—October—I attempted my first 100-miler. I had no idea what the heck I was doing. The course was rough with a lot of rock and flint. I was wearing my road running shoes. My feet were beaten up so badly. At mile 75—or there abouts—I quit or "DNF" (did not finish). I literally could not stand up anymore—the pain in my feet was so bad.

I was not going to give up…

The following year—February—I went down to Texas and ran in the Rocky Raccoon 100. I loved that race so much. The scenery. The people. The slower pace: a new thing because of my injuries. That one I did finish. My first 100-mile race—post accident—done! Less than two years after my accident.

There were a few more 100-milers in the next year or so. However, I started having a lot of abdominal problems due to the crash. So, more surgeries which included mesh to repair the damage from ribs that were cutting through the tissue. Unfortunately, my body didn't like the mesh; it started rejecting it, which meant more hospital visits. They would open me up, try different things, and stitch me up again. It was one thing after another. It seemed like every time I had new stitches, I got a new infection. It was crazy. I didn't think it would ever end.

Remember? I'm stubborn...

I started planning my races around the surgeries. I'd have a surgery scheduled. I knew I would be on antibiotics to keep any infection down. I'd time the race just right: I'd run the 100-miler on the weekend and show up ready for surgery on Monday. They would cut into my abs—most of the problems were in my abdominal area. My grand plan was to recover from the race and surgery at the same time. In about a month, I would do it all over again!

All this led to my first Slam race. A Slam race is a series of four 100-mile races—scheduled close to each other—and they add all the finishing times up together. The fastest time wins. In 2014 I completed—and won—my first Slam race.

That's when things really took off for me. I started running 12 to 15 100-mile races a year. Last year, I was scheduled for 36 100-mile races. Unfortunately, COVID shut most of them down.

Then, the day before Thanksgiving, I had a massive stroke. I guess a blood clot went through a hole in my heart and traveled up into my brain causing a stroke. This was the undetected heart defect I had since I was born.

It was a bilateral stroke, which meant both sides of my body were affected. I couldn't stand. I lost my vision and my ability to swallow. It was bad. Once again, the medical folks were preparing me for life in a wheelchair.

To make matters worse, all this happened during the pandemic. I had no visitors—not even my wife was allowed to see me. The rehab team was in contact with her, helping her—mentally and physically—get ready to care for someone who was completely disabled: a wheelchair, access ramps, grab bars, and other accommodations.

Again, I'm hardheaded...

After I stabilized from all the surgeries, I was sent to rehab. I was there for about a week. Some functions were slowly coming back, however, my legs just wouldn't work. I would try to crawl on the floor in my room. I tried to do push-ups from my knees—anything to stay active. The rehab staff would get angry with me because I wasn't following my doctor's orders.

The damage to my brain was in the medulla which controls essential involuntary functions such as breathing, circulation, and digestion. Consequently, my heart rate and lungs were also messed up. That has been devastating.

I don't think I have ever felt so desperate in my life... I worked and worked with the therapist to try and stand again. The doctors repeatedly conveyed that, "Some people recover; many people don't." They were trying to get me to prepare for the possibility that I may never walk again. They were not hopeful. I know they were trying to keep it real, and I appreciate that...

However, I would not quit. I worked relentlessly. I remember one particular day with the bars. I had worked to be able to stand up for eight seconds. Up until this point, when they'd let go of the gait belts, I would always fall over to my left side. My body literally couldn't hold itself up. Yet, that day I stood up without falling. Yes, it was only eight seconds. But it WAS eight seconds!

That day the rehab staff and I came to a loggerhead. They wanted me to go back to my room and rest. I wanted to stay and keep working at it. They insisted, "You need a break." Plus, they also explained that my "session was over" and "there aren't any therapists available to work with you right now."

As it happened, that day, there was a medical student in the room from Kansas University. He knew I was an ultra-runner, and he also saw how desperate I was. He offered to help. Thankfully, the team agreed; he stayed and we worked. Boy, did we work! We worked incredibly hard for 12 hours straight. The stroke really zapped my strength. It took every ounce of energy I had. By the end of that 12-hour period, I was walking! I stood and walked all in the same day. I was elated! After that, things really took off. I just got better and better.

In fact, I was walking so well, the insurance company refused to pay for any more rehab because I had "exceeded my treatment goals." Remember, they thought I would never walk again. Once the insurance company stopped paying, I was on the fast-track home.

As soon as I got home, I started outpatient rehab at a local clinic. They knew me and knew I was a big-time runner. I told them, "I can work on the walking. My big goal is to get back to running." Although, they weren't sure about how the insurance would work, they were up for the challenge. My rehab team was amazing. They set obstacles up off the floor for me to walk over, which was extremely hard due to my lack of coordination. Soon, they started taking me outside to a grassy area so I could try out my running skills. That way, when I fell—which I did a lot—it didn't hurt so badly. I did outpatient rehab for another 30 days. During that time, all the drills and exercises were 100 percent focused on getting me back to running. After rehab ended, I went home and continued to work on things myself. I kept trying. Working hard. In time, I had improved enough to return to work.

Two months after my stroke I felt ready to attempt my first 100-miler. I remember, it was super cold that day. Did I say how incredibly cold it was? The high was only five degrees. It was a tough 100-miler. Through mountains. Did I say how cold it was? I made it 53 miles. I discovered that when my brain got tired it just would not hold my body up anymore. I literally collapsed.

Later that year, I traveled to Louisiana, in much warmer weather, to run the Red Dirt Ultra, another 100-miler. I collapsed again. This time at mile 75. I am stubborn. Remember, I keep on trying...

More recently, in another attempt, I made it to mile 77 before I crashed. Total, race over, collapse. This time I used a Pacer. She let me take a 30-minute nap. I literally laid down on the trail and slept. It didn't help.

It's frustrating because I have completed all these races before. Easily. Some of them multiple times. It's something to do with the brain damage that I am still trying to figure out. It does seem that if I go slower and conserve my brain energy, I can finish. If I try to go back to my pre-stroke speed, it's a "no go." My brain can't tolerate it.

As I mentioned previously, the stroke damaged an area of the brain called the medulla. That area controls involuntary functions. Simple, everyday things we don't think about. Things we do automatically, like sneezing, for example—I haven't learned how to do that yet. However, I have relearned how to cough.

Of course, another involuntary function we don't think about is balance. Our ability to stand up and stay upright. I have had to relearn how to stand. Now, when I stand up to do anything—walking, running, taking out the trash—it takes an incredible amount of energy and concentration to keep my balance and stop myself falling over to my left. I have to think hard about the mechanics of it all, balancing, moving my feet, staying upright. As you can imagine, this has been incredibly difficult.

Before the stroke I took so much for granted. Standing up. Good balance. Walking. Running. That part of my brain is dead. It's true, the body is amazing. However, the body doesn't rebuild areas of the brain. This has been a difficult adjustment.

A stroke is not an injury that you heal or recover from. The body—bones, muscles, nerves—will rebuild themselves; the brain does not work like that. Yes, things in the brain can get a bit better. However, strokes are something you have to live with, manage, constantly adapt to—for the rest of your life.

*Please share a little about the role of nature in your healing process.*

Although I have finished six 100-milers post-stroke, I'm a good 12 hours slower than my pre-stroke times. For me, that's been devastating.

Before, I could show up at a race—without training—confident. Not worried about a thing. Today, clearly, that is no longer my reality. I am adjusting, trying to accept my limitations.

For sure, there's been some depression. What helps to get me out of that? Determination. When I feel down, I commit to training harder. That's just me. Even pre-stroke, when I had a failure. For example, a DNF—that would kick me into training harder.

I am also pretty competitive. Not so much against others, more with myself. Pre-stroke I had a back-to-back streak of 23 100-mile races. I was going for a record of 25 back-to-back races—then I had the stroke.

Setbacks make me work harder. Determination gets me through the tough times.

I love running and I love being outside. Trails are my biggest love. Currently, I am using dirt roads for training. That way I can still get out into the countryside with the trees, the sky, the earth beneath me. It's not the same as trails, but at least it's some connection with nature.

I feel like my body replenishes and heals better when I am outside. Nature restores me. I feel energized when I get out and run.

I am a big believer in keeping the blood flowing. Even when I am injured. Generally, the prescription for common injuries—like sprains or pulled muscles—is rest. Over a decade ago, I really looked into this. I don't do that. When I get an injury, within reason, I do something, even if it's mild exercise, to keep that area moving. The movement keeps the blood flowing through the injured area, which promotes faster healing.

Here's an example. I was flying down a very technical trail on a training run, leaping over all sorts of rocks, roots, and boulders. As I was going over a boulder, I misjudged it. I knew I was going to land short. In that split second, I decided to extend out my leg, in the hopes of reaching the next rock— to avoid crashing and falling. The guy I was running with, who was wearing headphones, heard a loud pop. My left hamstring snapped. I had a third-degree hamstring pull. Pretty serious. My whole leg turned black and blue, and the blood flowed all the way down into my calf. You can imagine the pain. Intense.

Anyway, I had a 100-mile race coming up in three weeks. With my leg the way it was, it didn't look good. That willpower kicked in. I was determined. I rolled the leg a lot. I exercised it as much as it felt comfortable. I kept it moving, encouraging that blood flow. In a week or so I was back to running. Three weeks later I completed that 100-mile race. Absolutely no issues. Generally, with a third-degree hamstring injury like that, you are out for three to six months. I am a big believer in the healing power of blood flow and movement.

From running so much, I sometimes get stress fractures in my feet. As a result, I have had broken metatarsals. I use the same movement/blood flow principles to stimulate the natural healing processes.

Here's another story. This is crazy... I was running the Tough Trail 100-miler. At mile 25, I fell hard, twisting my ankle badly. I jumped up, brushed myself off, and started running again. My ankle was particularly painful when I turned it from side-to-side. To compensate, I kept it straight and finished the race.

This race was part of a Slam Series. Two weeks later I had another 100-miler scheduled. I had been running just fine. No problems. About 71 miles into this second race, I started getting a horrible, sharp, nerve pain. Actually, first, I felt a tear in my calf muscle, the soleus muscle, a flat, broad muscle in the calf area. Then I felt searing pain, followed by a warm feeling; blood was flowing down. I wanted to finish the race. I kept running. The soleus got so inflamed it started hitting the post tubular nerve. It felt like a horrible, painful electrical shock.

At that point I was done running. I walked the final 29 miles to the finish line. Even with all that I came in under the 30-hour cut off time.

The next day I went to the doctor for the injury. They did several MRIs and discovered that when I twisted my ankle, I had actually snapped my fibula bone in half. I had no idea I had been running on an injury like that. The fibula is not a weight bearing bone. That's probably how I was able to push through. My mind and body adapted by keeping the ankle straight and blocking out the pain. In short, I had been running on a broken bone for about 170 miles—something I do not recommend.

Once again, I used the same method, movement, rolling, stimulating blood flow to repair this injury. With this injury—to keep the weight off my leg—I used a rowing machine. Rowing is my back-up plan, especially if I am healing a serious leg injury. With the rowing machine, I can baby the injured leg and adapt by using the healthy leg, my arms, back, and core muscles. I get a good bout of endurance training. And, more importantly, I keep that blood moving around my body. About three weeks after all that damage my leg healed.

As you can see, I have experienced a lot of injuries over my life. I've had to adapt and learn how to cope. My preferred method of healing is to harness the natural power within the human body. I'm not special. We are *all* hard-wired with these resources.

The human body is equipped with an incredible array of tools and mechanisms specifically designed for healing and repair. Blood flow is one example we can all relate to... The blood brings new cells, along with other healing compounds, to the wounded area. Bathing the injured area with all the good stuff. Then, on the way out of the area, the blood carries the damaged cells away for disposal. It's amazing!

As humans (and mammals), we have these systems for healing and managing pain naturally hard-wired into our bodies. As an endurance athlete, my brain and body has learned to harness these systems, which allows me to push through high levels of pain. However, again, I am not unique. We *all* have this ability.

Most people, when they get injured, seek medical attention, which, of course, is the right thing to do. The doctors, at least in traditional Western medicine, will usually suggest rest. In the past, I have also tried this method. Now, in comparison, "rest" seems like it takes forever for an injury to heal. For me, putting up with the pain and engaging the natural healing systems—within sensible limits, of course—and getting that fresh blood flow into the injured area is vital.

As for machines and medications, I do have a TENS unit, which uses low voltage electrical current to help stimulate blood flow and relieve pain. This can sometimes be helpful. Also, I never take ibuprofen or medications like that. If I need an anti-inflammatory, I go to nature's store house. Specifically, peppers which are packed with properties that reduce inflammation. When I am racing, I eat jalapeno peppers to combat or prevent inflammation. When possible, I prefer using natural remedies.

Another thing I want to point out is the power of repetition. Whether it's running, jumping rope, swimming—if you do it every day, your body will naturally adapt. The body will get better. Efficient. Stronger. The body's ability to adapt is another natural superpower.

I think that's what has happened with me. Before the stroke, I had the ability to run a 100-mile race pretty much every weekend. Back-to-back. When I reflect on my first ultra—it was so hard. So painful. Afterwards, I couldn't walk for a week. At the time, I could not imagine getting up and doing it all over again.

The human body is capable of so much more than we realize. The power of its systems. The performance of the chemicals it produces. The signs and signals it gives us. The body is incredible. I completely trust my body.

I try to turn to nature for all my medication and health needs. The only exception is the use of alcohol now and again. Some races allow alcohol. Occasionally, when I am running through the night, especially if it's cold, I will sip on a bit of whiskey. Just little sips, now and again. Alcohol is the only substance that bypasses the digestive system and goes right into the blood stream. A sip of Fire Ball helps keep me warm and gives me a quick boost of energy. Because I am metabolizing the alcohol so fast, I never get buzzed or that drunk feeling.

Other than the occasional sip of whiskey, I rely completely on the natural agents my body produces to manage everything. All the things nature gifted us with. Natural endorphins to manage pain. Natural adrenaline to keep me alert. Natural enzymes for digestion. We produce everything we need. I don't want to mess that up by adding artificial—over the counter—pain relievers, stomach pills, or energy boosters into my body. That's my opinion. It's what works for me...

As for nature, I have been incredibly fortunate. I have traveled and run in some spectacular locations. Just out of this world. I love Texas and Louisiana; they have those pine trees with the soft needles that smell so amazing. And the silvery green Spanish

Moss that cloaks many of the trees creates a mystical atmosphere.

I have also run in Appalachia, Colorado, and the Black Hills (South Dakota/Wyoming area)—all areas that are incredibly rich with nature. Then you have the desert, for example in Arizona or New Mexico, where there is a different beauty with the cacti, the dryness, and the vastness of the endless skies.

One of my favorite things to do is to run through trees. I love to watch them out of the corner of my eye. Peripheral vision. There is something exhilarating about physically moving among the trees coupled with the action of the trees whizzing by. It's probably primal. A subconscious thing. It feels completely natural. The cedars. The sights. The sounds. It's wonderful!

Have you ever run through pines? Their needles make a wonderfully soft foot bed, earthy aromas kick up with each step, and light patterns shift as the sun follows the arc of the sky.

I love Georgia. There the trails offer more of a jungle experience. It's hot and humid. I love the sound of the birds and insects. In Georgia, they also have lovely soft ferns that live among the trees. In the spring you can literally see the new, baby ferns unfurling, waking up alongside everything else.

I live in Kansas. Southern Kansas is a bit like the Ozarks: trees, rocky, technical, hilly. Central Kansas has an area that has an interesting mix of desert and prairie, with rolling hills, bluffs, woods, caves, and canyons threaded with ribbons of bright orange sand. In eastern Kansas the terrain changes again. There you find tall prairie grass and flint hills which make the terrain a bit more technical. Kansas is a mixed bag. Personally, I appreciate the variety.

### *Is there an experience in nature that stands out in your mind as particularly powerful?*

I have had a couple of things that stand out, particularly encounters with wildlife. While running in the Black Hills, I came across a mountain lion. I was in his territory. We kept our distance from each other. That stands out for sure.

I also remember one night, again running, this time through horribly dense fog. I ran straight into this big old buck deer. I didn't see him until the last second. We literally ran into each other—face-to-face. It all happened so fast. We were so close. I saw his huge, wide eyes glistening in my head lamp. I could make out a white underside, other than that, in that moment, I had no idea what I was facing. It took my brain a few seconds to register that I was face-to-face with a deer. It must have taken him a moment too. Startled—as fast as lightening, he turned and ran off, huffing and puffing and snorting back into the woods. That really caught me off guard…

The other experience that comes to mind was this time in Louisiana. I had been running all night. It was about 5 o'clock in the morning when I ran into a wild hog. It's not unusual to encounter wild hogs on the trail now and again. They usually turn tail and run off in the opposite direction. I didn't think much of it... However, this one was different. This hog was getting aggressive. Grunting, posturing, bristling up, preparing to charge. In a flash, I realized that she must be protecting babies somewhere close by. I was absolutely in her territory; she was not happy. We were in a standoff for a good 15 minutes. Thankfully, out of nowhere, a farm dog, probably hearing all the commotion, came running and chased her off. It took my heart a while to settle down after that one.

Snakes. I have also run into snakes, mostly water moccasins and rattlers.

I love the swamps and the bayous. The warmth. The humidity. The sounds. The wildlife. All so mysterious and beautiful in their own way. Running through this terrain feels like a welcome break from the single digit temperatures the Kansas winter serves up. T-shirt temperatures, with the warm sun on my face. Ahh... I cherish my time in these southern states.

As for beauty, in my opinion, Appalachia, Colorado, and the Rocky Mountains are stunning. The Appalachians—also known as the Appalachian

Mountains—are breathtaking. If I only ever got to run one more trail, it would be the Appalachian Trail. Running through those trees is one of my all-time favorite joys. Running through the night and experiencing the sun rising over those mountains, you feel the most powerful surge of natural energy.

Summer or winter, I always look forward to the sunrise. In the tough times, that's what I think about; imagine. That's what gets me through.

*What would you tell people who are currently experiencing what you went through?*

Since birth, I've had a rough time with my life and my health. Although I do get discouraged, I don't give up. I think that's vital.

Of course, I have felt depressed and discouraged. In general, I know it will only take a day or two for those feelings to pass. Then that determination kicks in. That's when I want—with every fiber of my being—to go out and crush it (whatever *it* is...).

Another thing I would say is, "Don't believe everything you hear or are told." If I had believed the doctors who told me, "You'll probably never walk again," or "Your running days are over," who knows where I would be today? When I hear things like that, it makes me want to prove them all wrong.

What I really want you to hear is, "Never give up!"

I learned this from a man I met during my first 50-mile race. We became fast friends. I'll always remember his advice, "When you're running a hundred miles, if things get bad—keep going—they will almost always get better." For the most part I have found that to be true. Of course, if you break a leg or something—that's different.

The fact is that running a hundred miles is a lot like life. You'll hit low points. You'll feel like quitting. If you can learn to push through the low points, your body and brain will find a way to overcome the adversity. You will hit another spurt of energy. Motivation. Willpower. Before you know it, your perspective will shift—for the better.

People quit too soon. Give your body a chance to adapt. Adjust. Overcome. In my experience, the body will figure out a way through. If it doesn't, then that's a sign to stop and take care of yourself.

Many times, early in a race, I'll notice an ache or a pain here or there. It could be my knee or my hip or my ankle. I know that if I keep moving those aches and pains usually disappear. Before long, I've forgotten all about them. By the time I've finished that hike, run, or walk it's like the discomfort has magically disappeared. Again, the body is truly amazing!

Here's another tip. Whatever you are trying to accomplish, keep practicing. The more you do, the better you will get. Don't worry about the numbers—

the distance, the time. Focus on building your mental stamina, "I'm going to finish this." Stay focused on your goal; over time, naturally, things will fall into place. Yes, there will be some discomfort. Remember, in time, your body and mind will adapt—it will get easier.

Through all this, the biggest lesson I have learned is to trust my body. Learn to understand and know your body, how it works, how it responds. Then whatever you are working toward—keep going. The human body is an incredible wonder of nature. Yes, for sure, at times you will be uncomfortable, but remember, like my friend told me years ago, "Don't give up!"

Unfortunately, with the stroke, the rules have changed. Life is not so simple. Due to the brain damage, after a certain point, I literally cannot stand up. As you can imagine, having no control of this basic, vital function has been devastating.

It's no longer about pain or pushing my body through things. Now, it's more about basic functional abilities. I am still experimenting, changing things up, getting more aggressive—and creative—with my training plan. I haven't and I won't give up.

If something isn't working for you, do a bit of research. Consider changing things up. Try different strategies. Adjust. As an ultra-runner, I have learned to adjust to all kinds to things. Weather. Heat. Storms. Cold. You name it!

You don't have to run a hundred miles to listen to your body. We all have an internal wisdom. Don't be afraid to adjust your plan, even if it is at the last minute. For example, when running, hiking, or walking in hot, humid weather, regardless of your "plans" adjust to the conditions. Slow down, through the afternoon heat, then pick-up your pace in the evening, when the temperatures have cooled off. The ability to adapt is another natural human superpower.

I've run in blizzards, monsoons, downpours, waist-high water, freezing cold, hail, high winds, mud—everything nature can throw at you. You push through and you finish. The circumstances of my life have taught me to not give up. I adjust. I overcome. I manage the discomfort. The feeling that comes after you have pushed through the brutal heat, the pain, the endless miles, hours upon hours on your feet—is indescribable. You feel on top of the world. You beat it! You pushed through and you beat it!

*What other tools have been helpful during your healing process?*

Although I am strong willed, I can't take all the credit. In all honesty, I'm not a fan of books. However, I like reading articles and blogs on the internet. That has been helpful.

Podcasts have been helpful too. Sometimes I will listen to a podcast while I am training. Right now, I am enjoying a podcast called *Ten Junk Miles*. It's lighthearted and easy to listen to.

*Run to Riot* is another podcast I like. I have been a guest on that show. I really like the guy that hosts it. We think a lot alike. I appreciate hearing inspirational stories from other runners. It helps keep me going when I am at those low points.

I enjoy these podcasts because they re-enforce what I am thinking or feeling. The message, "If it's not working for you, you have the power to change it," is a great example. When you connect with other people who are thinking, seeing, or experiencing the world the way you do—that helps cut through some of the isolation.

Sharing experiences and connecting with other runners who have the same problems has been helpful. I enjoy swapping information, tricks, and strategies with people too.

Generally, I am a bit of a lone wolf. I've never had a coach. I've learned everything by trial and error. I read, or listen, to other people's experiences, and sometimes that sparks an idea. I'll experiment, give it a try, see what works best for me, my body, and my circumstances. Again, it's tapping into that natural ability to adapt and change.

Also, remember that it's not so much about physical strength; it's more about mindset. Mentality. The mental ability to keep going and push through is vital. I have seen some exceptional athletes who lose it when they are pushed outside their mental comfort zone. Once discouragement sets in, they give up. Quit. Throw in the towel. Don't do that...

*From surviving to thriving: Tell me a bit about your life today.*

Well, this probably would have been a different conversation if I finished my last race. I was on a six-in-a-row streak. Recently, I have been in a low spot.

Currently, I'm on a learning curve. I am consuming a lot of information related to strokes and my disabilities. My current strategy is not working. So, I am doing something about changing that.

Since the stroke, life has been very frustrating. It's been hard to keep going. I am struggling to finish races within the 30-hour cut off time. Pre-stroke it was nothing to finish in around 22 hours. I am still two hours outside that time limit. Of course, I'm working on a new strategy.

My legs are still there. My tolerance for pain is still there. My willpower is still there. Once my brain gets tired, it just won't hold my body up. So, yes, it's been tough, frustrating, and hard to comprehend.

Right now, I am trying to work around my disability. On the right side of my body, my brain will not trigger my hamstring or my glute. These are vital muscles for running. To give you an example, pre-stroke my walking pace was around a 16-minute mile. Now, post-stroke—with fresh legs—I am walking at a 20-minute mile pace. That's it, no matter how hard I try. This is a result of my right leg not working correctly so I have to drag it along. On my left, the leg muscles are fine. However, the left side has coordination issues. If I'm on flat surfaces, it's not so bad. I still stumble because my foot droops. On trails, I don't have the coordination to navigate the rocks, roots, and other hurdles—it's really slowed me down. I have been avoiding technical trails. That said, I am training for a race in December. I've never run it before. The course is on horse trails. So, we'll see…

I have done a lot of research about strokes. Interestingly, I have a couple of friends—also runners—who have had strokes and still run. One of them just completed his first 100-miler last month. My other friend, Thomas Greene, has completed six 100-mile races, post-stroke. He's pretty popular. He runs with a stroller on rail trails to help him keep his balance. I tried that for a while and decided it wasn't for me. My goal is to get back to running traditionally.

I get to share a lot of my experiences with those guys. We have similar obstacles we are working on overcoming. We learn a lot from each other. That helps. The sense of community is so important.

The stroke has been the most challenging thing I have ever had to overcome. Even the motorcycle wreck was easier to deal with than this. Yes, I get discouraged. However, once I am done pouting and the negative thoughts have moved through, I feel better. More determined.

Recently, I have been pushing my body harder. It seems to be adjusting well—that feels good. I have had some successful runs in the past few weeks. In fact, right before we spoke, I had my fastest run since my stroke. Just four miles. But I *ran* the whole four miles—without taking a walk break! And I came in at under a 12-minute mile—slow—but fast for me. I am on a high right now, feeling excited, positive, hopeful. Tomorrow I'll try six miles and see how that goes.

### If you had one piece of sage advice to offer, what would it be?

My wife says I am the "hardest headed person" she knows. That's not just related to running—it's related to life. Whether it be a mechanical problem, a business concern, or a medical challenge—when I fail at something I go back and try and try again until I get it right. I guess I am naturally persistent. So, my sage advice? Simple. Be persistent. Push through. Trust your body. Never give up!

*Is there anything you want to add that we didn't cover?*

I'd like to remind people that we are all part of the natural world. Whatever the circumstance, we have these incredible bodies—capable of more than you can even imagine. We have access to a natural pharmacy. We produce all kinds of chemicals. Dopamine for motivation. Adrenaline for managing pain. Other chemicals that naturally heal, repair, and restore.

Running has been my savior… A long time ago, when I was first getting into running, on the weekends, I would get up at three in the morning and head out for a 20- or 30-mile run. On the weekdays I would be up and out for a ten-mile run. Back home. Shower. Then off to work.

I feel so good after coming in from being outdoors. All that physical movement. All that oxygen. All those endorphins. On the days I don't run, my mood suffers. I feel more down. Depressed. Blah. In short, running is my life. I am determined to keep going…

———

# JANIE BAXTER

Hiker—healing from a painful childhood and relationship trauma—
rebuilding her life through walking, nature, and spirituality

*"Slowly, I started to regain my sense of confidence. I began feeling stronger. Empowered. As I continued to cope with the fallout from my marriage, the divorce, and my childhood..."*

– Janie Baxter

**JANIE AND HER STORY** touched my heart... You know, as infants, we don't get to choose how, where, or to whom we show up. We hope for the best, yet we all ultimately know it's a crap shoot. Luck of the draw. From the beginning—not a hint of complaint—Janie describes a challenging set of circumstances: addiction, anger, money struggles, complex blended family dynamics, abandonment, pain, and suffering. If you are thinking, "Wow! That's a lot," you are right. Janie has endured a lot.

Janie guides us through childhood, her turbulent teen years, which tumbled right into an unhealthy relationship, and marriage, resulting in over 16 years of escalating anger, abuse, and trauma.

As I listened to Janie's story, I witnessed her immense courage, her innate wisdom, and her fearlessness. Janie candidly recounts the many painful twists and turns of her healing journey through trauma, anxiety, and a Post-Traumatic Stress Disorder (PTSD) diagnosis. A journey which started with her decision to "get real" with her thoughts, her feelings, and her reality. Gradually, through walks, solitude, time in nature, radical honesty, and her growing spirituality—glimmers of healing, hope, and recovery began to shine through.

Thank you, Janie, for offering your story... Through these words, I hope you, dear reader, will be encouraged, inspired, driven to discover your own glimmer of hope and healing—whatever that may be for you. With honor, respect, and deep gratitude...

### Janie B

*Tell me a bit about you and your background.*

Childhood was challenging. I'm one of four children in my immediate family, and one of 11 if you count my step- and half-siblings. My father was an alcoholic; motivated by the prospect of jail, he quit drinking. He's now in recovery. He quit drinking because he faced jail time. He didn't subscribe to Alcoholics Anonymous (AA) or anything like that—he relied on willpower to keep him sober.

My mom worked hard. She kept up appearances. She baked cookies, picked out thoughtful gifts, attended our school events, and made sure we were clean and fed. However, underneath the surface, my mom struggled with her own mental health concerns. She kept it to herself. She was good at hiding it, keeping everything inside. Until, one day, she had a breakdown.

Dad had a temper. He was careful not to break things; intimidation was his preferred practice. As a kid I remember Dad telling us that he had eyes everywhere, that people were watching us, "So we'd better be where we said we'd be and with who we said we would be with." I can hear him now, "Don't make me lose my temper," was a common start to a difficult evening.

My dad was also a skilled negotiator—impossible to argue with. He would talk circles around me, tying me up in knots, until I had no defenses left. Of course, in my family, any expression of emotions was disallowed—a sign of weakness, which was swiftly dealt with.

Middle school hit, and things got worse. My mother met another man, and she left—abandoning us for a new life and another family. My youngest sibling wasn't even in school yet.

Predictably, my father relied heavily on me to take care of the kids and him. I did my best. I cooked. I cleaned. I copied Mom's recipes. I sewed and mended. At one point, I even contemplated dropping out of school to care for my youngest brother. So much responsibility. So many expectations and so little agency over my life.

Consequently, much of my childhood was spent caring for others. Over time, the natural world became the place I could find a bit of peace and comfort. The outdoors became the place I felt cared for. Nurtured. I remember a big cottonwood tree in our front yard. In between the chores and the childcare, I would climb up to my favorite branch and just sit in stillness. Sometimes, I would watch the sunset or listen to the leaves rustle. Often, I would cry and speak to the tree as if it could hear my grievances.

Other times I would hop on my bike, head down a country road, and work hard to pedal away my anger and frustration. Pretty soon, I'd find myself out in the middle of nowhere surrounded by beautiful fields. One day, out of the blue, I remember a goat wandering up to me—so curious— that little guy totally made my day!

When families are in survival mode there is typically little time, or energy for the outdoors. That said, as kids, one thing we were allowed to do was choose how we wanted to celebrate our birthdays. Every year, my request was always the same—to spend some time outside, specifically a visit to Split Rock and Gooseberry Falls up on the north shore of Lake Superior. Even though that was a long time ago, I still remember the feeling, the sense of peace that came from being out in nature.

Thanks to my church youth group, I also got to experience camping. During the summer, the church would pack us up and take us on an overnight camping adventure. Sometimes, if we were lucky, we'd go for a whole weekend. I can't tell you—at that age and that time in my life—how incredibly freeing it felt to be outside, in the woods, with the trees, and the sound of the water nearby.

In nature my body could exhale. My lungs could relax enough to take a full breath again. The sunsets, the smell of a freshly cut field, the hum of the bumblebees. The tranquility of deer grazing or the bob of the white underside of a rabbit's tail would feel like a brief reprieve. Magically transporting me—for a moment—out of the pain of my circumstances. Those were special times I still hold on to…

Nature became the only place where I could let my feelings show without consequence. With nature on my side, I could find just enough sanity—strength—to face returning home, to walk in the door and slip into my room, avoiding the evening's inevitable confrontations.

*Diving into the tough topic, tell me a bit about your personal journey/experience.*

I shared a little about my early childhood above. As you can imagine, I was desperately unhappy and could not wait to leave home. Predictably, I met a man. We quickly married. I should have been wiser about choosing a spouse. Looking back there were warning signs, red flags, of course. I was young, my view of what a healthy relationship looked like and felt like was colored by my childhood experiences.

One day I will never forget is the day he planned to propose. I was sick and craving an orange soda. I asked if we could run through the drive thru. He was reluctant, but we went. As the bubbly orange liquid hit my stomach, I started feeling really nauseous. I opened the car door and wretched my guts up. He got incredibly angry. He blamed me for throwing up, yelling, "I should have never ordered the drink." Somehow, because I got sick, I "ruined" the plans *he* had of proposing to me. I remember feeling tired, weak, and emotionally exhausted.

The second time he proposed wasn't much better. It was wintertime. I didn't have a car, so I walked to work. That day, because the weather was so crummy, he offered to pick me up after work. Well, I waited and waited—he never came. It was nighttime and well below zero; fighting slippery sidewalks covered with inches of thick, heavy Minnesota snow, I started walking.

He eventually showed up about a block from my house saying "he forgot." I was mad, and he knew it; he suggested we go out to dinner to "make up for it." "Fine," I thought. I quickly changed out of my work clothes, threw on a pair of jeans and a flannel shirt. As I came into the living room, he said, "You're not to going to wear that, are you?!" "Geez," I thought, "You lack compassion for me on every level and now you're telling me how I should dress?" That night, we went out to dinner, he proposed, and I said, "Yes…"

Back then, in some odd way, all this felt normal. As a child, I had learned to be quick to forgive and accept excuses. A part of me was optimistic, hopeful for a man he was never going to become. Plus, I held the belief that—for better or worse—the years you were married were a badge of honor. I spent 16 years battling the vicious cycle of abuse. He was charming. He would blowup. He would apologize and promise to behave differently. Things would be okay for a while. Something would set him off and it would happen all over again.

It got worse after we had children. Everything became a target for his anger. My labor pains, the children crying, a messy kitchen were all grounds for him throwing and breaking things. Toys on the floor became excuses to punch holes in the walls. In time, the messy parts of everyday family life became a minefield. I tried hard to stay ahead of his temper. I'd anticipate, plan, and scheme, "What could possibly inconvenience him?" "How could I ensure a peaceful evening?" "What could set him off?" I would clean the kitchen, rush to put the toys away, and frantically pick up the house. Of course, it didn't help. He'd find something. He would yell, and blame, and point fingers, "You made me this way. This is your fault. If only you would…" I remember feeling like a complete failure, like I was responsible for his anger, his outbursts, his rage.

As I mentioned, he was charming. Like many abusers, he knew all the right words. He was also skilled at being both the perpetrator and the victim. He could inflict harm, neglect my feelings, and still find a way to get me to comfort him and take the "blame" for causing him harm. Having a voice and standing up for myself resulted in him breaking down, hating himself, promising to change, and desperately begging for forgiveness. It was so painful, he so wanted to be cared for but wasn't willing—or didn't know—how to care for others. Eventually we divorced.

As I navigated the divorce and custody proceedings, nature became a priority for me. I was facing a broken marriage, an empty house, the children were often gone visiting their father or out with friends. The silence. The stillness. The anxiety. I was worried about their safety, their wellbeing, and my own mental and physical health. I felt absolutely shattered.

During this period, a part of me knew that I had to start spending some time taking care of myself. With this realization came questions like, "What do I want?" "What do I like?" "What is important to me?" Of course, these inquiries led to bigger reflections such as, "Who am I as a person?" and "What do I want my life to look like?" At the time, I fully identified as a wife, a mother, a caretaker. Thinking about me and what I might want for my life was completely new territory for me. I have to tell you—I was terrified.

*Please share a little about the role of nature in your healing process.*

I remembered a friend growing up. She had this horse that would hold its breath and puff out his stomach every time you wanted to saddle up. We'd run that horse around in circles. He would work up such a sweat, until he had no choice but to let go and breathe naturally. Only then could we get that saddle on and ride.

That sense of holding my breath resonated deeply with me. I felt a lot like that horse. I knew I had to work up a sweat and break down my barriers. I had to get honest with myself. Real with my thoughts. Real with my feelings. Real with God...

First, it started with small hikes. Local state parks. Usually alone. It was quiet. Slowly, I could begin to breathe. I am a person of faith. Out in nature, I could pray aloud. My circumstances didn't necessarily change, nothing was solved. Yet, somehow, time in nature, the process of working up a sweat, and starting to slow down, began to soothe some of my wounds. The barriers, the layers of pain, the loss, the hurt started to melt—just a little. In nature I could share whatever I needed to. Something—God, Mother Nature—was listening, and I was beginning to heal.

In time, I began to regain my sense of confidence. I started feeling stronger. More empowered. As I continued to cope with the fallout from my marriage, the divorce, and my childhood, I felt incredibly grateful to have this time and space.

By this time, the symptoms of anxiety and Post-Traumatic Stress Disorder (PTSD) were part of my everyday life. The natural world provided a space where I could feel calm, safe. Nature helped take the edge off the trauma. Nature became my beacon for hope. Something to look forward to… It was as if my body knew when it needed to get outdoors. It's funny, even my children began to recognize my need to get outside. They would say, "Mom, I think you're due for a walk."

At this point, I've hiked every state park in Minnesota. Now, I am working my way through the Superior Hiking Trail—walking little segments at a time. I'm nowhere near my goal, and that's okay. For me it's not about time and miles; it's more about soaking up every moment and healing.

I hike year-round. I've learned to adapt to the weather, to be prepared. Learning about and having the right gear has been a fun part of the process. People at the local stores have been so helpful and generous in sharing their time and their knowledge.

That's another change: for the first time in a while, I am enjoying the sense of community. Connecting with other people who also celebrate the natural world, especially other backpackers. It's a different world. People are interested in sharing what they've learned. They want to give you tips. There's freedom in conversation that you don't find on the street.

In nature I feel like I can let go, release the mind, open the body—it's hard to verbalize. In nature my body has the freedom—or maybe it's just more willing to do things that it doesn't want to do when I'm at home or sitting at my desk.

In nature I can be myself. My body can be challenged. There's something powerful about physically moving through the natural world. My muscles, my lungs, my legs all work so much harder when I'm out on the trail. I love the way I feel after a long day of hiking. I am hungry. Meals are tastier, and I connect with the food nourishing my body. There is a wonderful sense of peace and calm. I worked hard. I overcame obstacles. I feel accomplished.

Through my connection with nature, I have learned to just be... The comfort that comes from the reality that in this moment not one soul on this planet needs anything from me. That feels amazing! A huge relief. I am simply here. Connected. Safe. At home under the big sky, on this earth, feeling the breeze— brings me a wonderful sense of peace and calm.

And the sights, the sounds, the smells... Oh my gosh, frogs! Frogs are one of my favorite creatures. When I start hearing the frogs croaking, or hear other animals, I stop still, and a huge smile lights up my face; knowing there are little critters nearby fills me with wonder.

In nature things are constantly changing. I may have walked a particular path a thousand times, yet I always notice things I have missed or how things have changed. I love that feeling of curiosity: What is up around the next hill? What will I see at the top of the next vista?

Revisiting my favorite parks during different times of the year is another way I connect with nature and the diversity nature brings. Here in Minnesota, we have four distinct seasons. Each season has its unique joys, challenges, and beauty. Even winter. Believe me, I hate being out in the cold, yet I've discovered that nature in winter has its own splendor and magic. For me, each season is filled with fond memories. I know that sounds wild, but that's the truth. Even winter. Especially, in winter, I love the quiet. The stillness. The peace. Often, I am the only human around for miles and miles.

A while back, I had a horse-riding accident. I ended up in the emergency room with a traumatic brain injury (TBI) and a long road to recovery. Consequently, my memory is a bit shaky. To compensate, when I am out on the trail, I take a lot of photos. Pictures help remind me of the beauty and the diversity. Through photos I can recreate that deep sense of deep connection I have with the natural world.

The other day I was writing, I didn't post it or anything, but the gist of it was about an experience I had hiking where it felt like a worship service—the oaks were standing tall and proud for the reading of the gospel. The frogs were singing in response to the psalms. The crows were preaching. The flowers were giving their offerings of beauty, color, light—so much emotion…

I think it's the spiritual part of me that makes me stop and pause. Notice. Look around. Pay attention. Once I'm away from the stresses and strains of life, my mind begins to slow down. I start to see that my connection with the natural world is part of something much bigger. Instead of being a consumer—wrapped up in efficiency and productivity—I feel aligned. A part of something vast, something infinite, something limitless.

*Is there an experience in nature that stands out in your mind as particularly powerful?*

That's a great question. I think all my experiences in nature have impacted me. In some way, even the drive to the trail head and the anticipation of stepping out of the car. I notice myself breathing deeper. My body relaxing.

This feeling is particularly powerful in the Boundary Waters, a region of wilderness that straddles the border between Canada and the United States just west of Lake Superior. I've been going there since my kids were little. I started taking them in the winter, which in hindsight, was crazy.

Our church offered a winter camp as a thank you. A retreat of sorts with time to connect with our own families after a busy season of teaching, mission trips, and church community events.

To get to the island in the wintertime, you had to cross a frozen lake—on foot—with all your gear (which, admittedly, seems really crazy with small children who were still in diapers). "Yeah, let's go into the wilderness, a place nobody goes, where it's 40 below zero. Yes, we could all perish, but that's cool. Right?"

Along with time for family, there was also space for personal solace. Time where I could decompress, enjoy nature, stretch my body and mind, and soak up the beauty of it all.

As the kids got older, we went on canoeing trips together. The camp would provide a guide (which, I was thankful for). Having a guide made that part of the world easier and safer for us to access. The conversations we had about the sun setting and the moon rising. About the stars and the night sky. About knowing, seeing, and being a part of the natural rhythms of life. Boy! Those times were invaluable.

When you leave your watch, your phone, and your devices behind and you begin to unhook from artificial time constraints, pretty quickly our bodies begin to rediscover their natural rhythms: when to eat, when to sleep, when to work, when to play. Instinctively, you start waking up with the dawn, eating when you are hungry, getting ready for bed as the sun goes down. I even learned to predict when those pesky black flies and mosquitoes would start showing up for their evening feast.

Throughout the day we worked hard—paddling, paddling, paddling. We saw incredible wildlife like eagles tending their babies, and loons—water birds that come right up to your canoe. I pushed my mind and body to do things I didn't think I was capable of. We all worked together. At the end of the day, I felt incredibly satisfied.

My kids feel this too… We do a lot of traveling together. After the divorce, I gave them a map of the United States and said, "Pick a spot and we'll go explore." We've done that every year. We know how to travel together and how to get things done. They know everybody contributes and shares a piece of the responsibility for the community—you're cooking tonight, you're doing dishes, you're helping to set up the tents—we all pitch in. We cherish that time, maybe because it's so unlike what our "normal time" looks like? The natural world has become a part of who we are as a family.

*What would you tell people who are currently experiencing what you went through?*

Looking back, anxiety has been a part of my life since childhood. Of course, it got worse during my marriage—crushing anxiety which culminated in frequent panic attacks. I began to think there was something horribly wrong with me. I didn't understand what my body was doing; I couldn't trust it. It took a while for me to understand what was happening. I thought I was handling things. I thought I was being strong, taking care of my children, and being a supportive wife. Over time, the anxiety and the trauma started affecting my health. That's when I sought therapy; unfortunately it didn't quite take... Not every therapist is the right therapist at the right time. I assumed that because I was going to therapy, that we, as a couple, would figure stuff out—together.

I wish I would have pursued things a little differently. All the stress was beginning to affect my health. I recall a time where I had these headaches and a tingling in my scalp that just wouldn't go away. I saw a neurologist. Unfortunately, he had the worst bedside manner. He said, "Yeah. I think this is all in your head. You need to get that figured out." I was so offended, but honestly, it was probably the best thing he could have said. It made me stop and think, "Maybe this isn't physical; is there something else I should be doing for myself?" It was a jolt of reality. I'm thankful for that. Please, listen to your body. Take notice of any physical signs that could be impacting your health (headaches, joint pain, stomach issues).

Finding the right therapist is also important. Be open to trying a few; therapeutic fit is vital. Most therapists are helpful, but just like cars, there's a lot to choose from. Not every car is going to be the right fit for your needs. If you are seeing a therapist and feeling that you're not receiving the benefits or making the progress you were hoping to make, it's okay to look for another provider. Remember, it's not necessarily anything against the therapist. Sometimes it's just not a good fit. It took me a while to find somebody (a therapist) who could help me navigate some of the more difficult, deeper conversations. Discussions that were never broached in my initial counseling experience.

Dealing with icky, ugly, uncomfortable things is an important part of the healing process. It doesn't mean the yucky stuff magically vanishes. However, it does mean you're better able to manage it when it does come up. You get to be in the driver's seat. Of course, the PTSD and the anxiety still pop up now and again, but they are no longer in control. That's a huge relief. I've learned a lot through the therapy process.

Another thing I would suggest is self-care— making time to care for yourself. I had to learn this too. When part of your identity is so used to taking care of other people, the concept of self-care can feel uncomfortable or even selfish. Learning how to care for yourself is another building block in the healing process. In many ways I had to deconstruct and then rebuild my identity. Through this process, I learned to be more present, accept who I am, and create new ways of showing up in my life.

Before, I blended into the background, enmeshed in the roles of wife, mother, daughter. Today, I'm no longer a tag-a-long, "Oh you are so-and-so's mom, or so-and-so's spouse, or so-and-so's daughter." Yes, I am a mother and a daughter. And, yes, I was a spouse. Today, I stand for myself, even in relationships with other humans. Through this journey—nature, therapy, healing—I have learned how to be me.

*What other tools have been helpful during your healing process?*

Building a sense of community has been important. I needed to feel more comfortable with being uncomfortable. Once I started to feel like, "It's

okay, I can do this; I am curious about this too…"
then I could relax a little.

I started to push myself a little by posting
pictures of my adventures on Facebook. People
began commenting and asking questions. They
were curious—interested—about locations, trails,
trail conditions, and what to expect. Pretty soon I
became the person they'd go to for information and
questions like, "I'm looking for a park with such
and such features, what would be a good option?" I
had a knowledge base I hadn't had before. It made
me laugh. I didn't feel like I was doing anything
remarkable. I'm not an extreme athlete or an
expert. I just like to wander. I enjoy the
connections I make with people. For the first time
in a long time, I felt encouraged. Supported.

Online groups have also been helpful. I
connected with the Superior Lake Hiking group on
Facebook. A wonderful group where people are
welcome to say, "Hi! I want to do this. I have no
experience, what's your recommendation?" People
are excited to share their experiences. There's no
sense of criticism, "Oh, you don't know what
you're doing, blah, blah, blah…" No, there's none
of that. I am very grateful for these groups and
communities.

I love books… I am in seminary school so I read
a lot of books about spirituality. I highly
recommend Jan Richardson's poetry and anything

by Mary Oliver. I love *Guerrillas of Grace* by Ted Loder and writers like Parker Palmer and Henri Nouwen. I remember there was even a little devotional I picked up at Yosemite Park which included some sayings from John Muir. My spiritual growth, along with my emotional and physical healing, has evolved organically through self-exploration, reading, prayer, and lots of time out in the natural world.

*From surviving to thriving: Tell me a little bit about your life today.*

Because I spent so long surviving, I just didn't realize how exhausted my mind and body were. For me, thriving is the ability to breathe again. One of my children, after his father left the home, said, "You know, I don't have to walk on eggshells, worrying about accidentally setting Dad off. Mom, I can breathe again. I know I am not the problem." I think that was also very true for me. I no longer feel like I am a problem.

To begin to thrive, people—families—need a sense of safety, peace, trust, and a confidence that everything is workable. Now when I go to sleep at night, I am not worrying, anxious, scared, or wondering if everybody is going to be okay. I feel healthier and see my kids happier—physically, mentally, spiritually. That feels good.

Self-care and time in nature created space for us to have conversations and share thoughts. Sometimes we take care of ourselves with our therapist, other times we go to the gym, sometimes we get out on the trail: it's all good. Interconnected, like a house of cards, each need connecting with another. If one card pops out of place, the whole thing falls apart. By tending to my spiritual, my physical, and my emotional needs, I know I am operating at my best. Yes, on a day-to-day basis, crap still happens, but it's not the end of the world. A difficult day doesn't have the soul-sucking impact it used to have.

### *If you had one piece of sage advice to offer, what would it be?*

One of the things I was concerned about—because of my faith—was that if I chose to step out of this marriage, I was disappointing God. I remember someone saying to me, "You are a beloved child of God. If you think that this doesn't make God angry, it does. He is pissed. He loves you. He doesn't intend for you to be treated this way. How does staying in this relationship bring honor to God?" Those words, that question, gave me a sense of freedom. They helped me see how God loves me. How I fit into His larger picture. Instead of worrying about what was happening with my marriage, it gave me the courage, the confidence, the clarity to say, "I put the work in. There are habits here… Things have been addressed and things are not changing. It's in my and my family's best interest to remove myself. That doesn't mean I don't love that person or that I don't love God." I know that God will still love me and consider me a precious child—regardless.

### Is there anything else you want to add that we didn't cover?

Yes, there are two more things I would like to share. One is the expression, "The best views are on the other side of the hill." For me this has been so true. My life, although it hasn't been easy, is so different today. If you are afraid or uncertain, I encourage you to lean into the discomfort and get the help and the support you need. Know that, on the other side of the mess, there is hope.

Lastly, whether it's five minutes or five miles, young, old, fast, slow, in shape or out of shape—it doesn't matter. Get outdoors. Get moving. Nature isn't just some place deep in the woods nor is it an exclusive club—it's open and accessible to everyone. Give it a try! What do you have to lose?

———

# DR. BETTY HOLSTON SMITH

Teacher, coach, ultra-runner—a lifetime of healing from segregation, discrimination, obesity, and harmful medical advice—at 81 years old, Dr. Betty has rebuilt her life though education, movement, and immersion in the natural world

*"I give credit to my mother and father for the way they valued education and encouraged us. For the freedom we had within our home. And I give credit to those massive, beautiful, virgin woods..."*

– Dr. Betty Holston Smith

LAST, BUT CERTAINLY NOT LEAST, is Dr. Betty—an amazing human being. Witnessing and sharing her story has been an honor. Have you ever walked through a stand of giant redwood trees or summited a mountain peak? Then maybe you can relate to the sense of awe, wonder, and gratitude such experiences can evoke. That best describes how a part of me felt...

Her wisdom, her deep connection with the natural world, and her effervescent energy were palpable. So much so that I recognized that sticking to the proposed "talking points" would diminish her story, interfere, and limit her flow. Once our conversation began, intuitively, I decided to get out of the way. Consequently, what follows is the unabridged version of Dr. Betty's journey.

On reflection, it seems that my instinct served me well. In our back-and-forth post interview "thank you" correspondence, Dr. Betty shared, "I've never had the opportunity to do this with anyone over all these years. [People] are always interested in one part of my story or another. They want to know [about] vegan eating or organic eating or running or whatever—but never my whole story. The entire me. I really appreciate you doing this…" (Personal email.)

Dr. Betty, your encouragement to eat chia seeds daily, to set guilt-free boundaries with family and friends, and to find ways to embody nature in every aspect of my life has been invaluable—thank you!

In the following pages, Dr. Betty shares her daily routine along with her secrets to longevity. I hope you too will discover a couple of threads or actionable steps that you can incorporate into your healing journey.

## Dr. Betty

*Tell me a bit about you and your life.*

My parents came from Georgia and Tennessee. Married very young, they made their way to the Washington metropolitan area, settling down in a little town in Maryland called Chevy Chase. An affluent area, where back then, and even today, a lot of the movers and shakers in the country lived.

I grew up surrounded by affluence. If you were not white, you didn't live in Chevy Chase on your own. Wealthy families lived in Chevy Chase because it was close to Washington, DC. We lived on a little street called Hawkins Lane. I call it a street. More accurately, it was a dirt road, there to house the service workers. I'm Black. Everybody on the street was Black—Black families working hard in mostly service jobs.

I was one of six children. My parents, not traditionally educated, were wise and understood the value of education. Growing up our house was known as the "homework house." My mother and father made sure we had everything we needed—pens, paper, encyclopedias, typewriters—to support our education.

The kitchen table was our hub for learning. Although there was a good ten years between my oldest and youngest siblings, everybody had homework. My mother would be there with us. Helping. Guiding. Encouraging. There was a time, a place, an expectation.

As we studied, my father was always close by. As he sat in his favorite chair, he listened to what was going on around the table. He was the one to say, "I think they need more paper," or "It's time for new encyclopedias," or whatever we needed.

His reward was report card time. We had to line up, in front of his chair, according to age. My father would sit and study every report card. He provided encouragement. Compliments. And, at least for me, the message that, "I could do better if I worked harder." "Always do your very, very best" was my parents' mantra. Once you've done your very, very best there's nothing more you can do. Work hard and do your best became ingrained in my brain. It was the only thing I knew how to do.

Consequently, I work really hard at everything. I cannot take on a job, a career, a chore, a run—whatever—without doing my very, very best. People tell me, "Betty, you go way beyond what you need to do..." Yes, that's true. And my mind goes right back to that homework table.

Life for us was totally segregated. Totally. I remember having to go to Washington, DC, to find products for our hair. Our skin. Nothing accommodated us locally. As a child, I knew we were segregated. However, I didn't know we weren't rich.

Growing up, I always had questions about segregation—especially once I got into school and started learning about the Constitution and the Bill of Rights. I'm going to stay with my own experience here... In Chevy Chase I was brainwashed in such a way that, for me, the messages I received in childhood felt 100 percent true. I *knew* that because of the color of my skin I was less worthy than white people. Less human. Undeserving. These were the beliefs I grew up with. The way I saw myself. My truth.

I'm 81 years old. About 25 years ago I realized that if I had been brainwashed to such an extent, then white people had been equally brainwashed to believe that they were put on this earth to be served by Black people. This shift in my awareness opened up a whole new perspective and understanding about white people, segregation, and freedom.

Okay, back to growing up... Our home on Hawkins Lane was surrounded by virgin woods and lots of nature. Of course, due to segregation, there were no playgrounds for Black children. So, the woods became our playground. We did everything in those woods. We climbed trees. We ran for miles. We made sling shots in the summer and enjoyed sleigh rides in the winter. No matter the season, the woods were a magical place full of wonder, learning, and adventure. Our outdoor home, where we felt safe and happy.

During those formative years, I developed a deep knowledge of the natural world. I knew nature's patterns. I could predict the first hint of spring and the arrival of delicate wildflowers. I knew the trees. All the shapes, colors, sizes. How they were all different yet all interconnected. How they adapted to the sunlight, to the shade, to the seasons. I learned to tell the time by noticing the position of the sun in the sky. All day, every day, I internalized nature's wisdom. Nature became a good friend. I could count on her. She never discriminated.

We, as kids, would be gone for hours and hours. Our days would be filled. Active. Spent piling leaves, building structures from branches, and exploring insects. I particularly remember the June bugs. As kids, we would tie a string around a June bug's legs, stand in one spot and go around and around and around. That June bug would be flying at the end of that string. We were careful not to cause harm. Once we let them go, they would fly away. Those poor June bugs.

I'm not a real bug or worm person. One day, a butterfly landed right on my shoulder. I was elated. So happy—in that moment—to be friends with a butterfly.

The woods were perfect. A wise teacher. Safe. Friendly. Welcoming.

Our little lane was also home to an abundance of trees: hickory nut, black walnut, peach, pear, and apple trees. There were grape arbors and all kinds of vegetables: cucumbers, radishes, squash, peppers, and tomatoes. What's more, we had access to it all. When we were out all day playing, we never went hungry.

Growing up, church was important... After Sunday school, my mother would buy a package of (I don't know if people will remember this...) Necco wafers. The wafers came in a little package. The actual wafers were small, maybe twice the size of a quarter. All different flavors and colors. My mother would divide the wafers among the six of us, which meant we probably got two or three each. Every now and then, again, after church, we would get ice cream cones. Now, that was a real treat! That was the extent of our "junk food."

Our food came from the outdoors. Apples. Walnuts. Peaches. I knew exactly when everything was ready to eat. As kids, we would instinctively monitor nature's progression. In the springtime, we would look for the blossoms that would soon become the inside of the fruit. Did you know peach trees have the most beautiful flowers? I remember, watching and waiting and watching and waiting, then, all of a sudden, magically, a tiny peach would appear. We knew not to eat those. We knew we had to wait. We also knew we wouldn't have to wait that long until we could grab a juicy peach or apple or pear from the trees.

Needless to say, we grew up eating lots of raw fruits and vegetables and nuts. Did you know that the shells of walnuts and hickory nuts are incredibly hard? Back then we had no nutcrackers. If we wanted what was inside, we had to figure out how to crack open those tough little shells. It was my job to scout out the right rock. It takes precision, determination, and creativity to crack a walnut. The tools? Two rocks and a pin. We would position one rock on the ground and place the nut on the rock. The force of the second rock cracked the nut. The pin was used as a pick to gather the fruit after the nut was cracked. I remember repeating this process over and over again until those little nuts conceded.

We rarely came in for lunch, much to my oldest sister's chagrin. She would make peanut butter sandwiches and line them up in neat little rows, patiently waiting for us to come home. Sometimes, we were late. Often, we didn't show up at all. Either way, we never went hungry.

So, that was my childhood... Lots of time in the woods, surrounded by nature and the wonders of the natural world. We learned to adjust to the seasons as they came and went. We knew spring always followed winter. That spring brought a sense of hope and promise of new life.

In 1954, when schools were desegregated, I was 13. My father decided to let desegregation take hold for a while before making any decisions about our education. In the interim, he insisted that his children continue to be segregated in our local school district. At that time there was a Black university and a white university. My oldest sister was attending the Black university of Maryland. My next oldest sister, who was in the 12th grade, was a student at the Black high school in Rockville, Maryland.

Back then, all Black children were educated in Rockville, the county seat of Montgomery County. School buses would pick up all the kids and bus them to school. For many, including my sister, this meant a two-hour bus ride before and after school.

Fast forward to 1956... My father had given it two years for desegregation to settle in. At that time, I was ready for 10th grade. He decided I was going to be one of the first Black children to "help" integrate the 10th grade of Bethesda Chevy Chase Senior High School (BCC). At the time, BCC was home to 3,500 affluent white students. Recall that Chevy Chase is located just outside Washington, DC.

Also, remember that I am coming from Rockville, Maryland, where Black people were bussed. There was no kindergarten for Black children. My elementary school was a small wooden building with a pot-belly stove. We had substandard everything: resources, teachers, books, supplies, education. Our furnishings and supplies came, well-worn, from the white schools in the area. Despite these barriers, I developed a love for learning. This, I am proud to say, was reflected in my report cards (with As and a few Bs here and there...).

As mentioned, in the summer of 1956, it was time for high school. Located in downtown Bethesda, Maryland, BCC was a multi-floor brick building which sat way back off the street. The first day of school, my mother dropped me off. There were no "meet and greets." No orientations. Nothing. My father was adamant, "This is the best public high school in America. You need to take advantage of that education." Of course, he was absolutely right. However, in my head I did not deserve to be in a school with white kids. Remember, I believed I was defective—not a complete human.

Here I am. Walking down the sidewalk. An A student. I remember hugging a brand-new notebook close to my chest. Feeling half human. As I look around, I see a sea of kids out in the front of the school. Greeting each other. Smiling. Laughing. Catching up on their summer news, trips, and vacations. As I walked down that sidewalk the entire world became silent. All those warm smiling eyes were directed right toward me. Looking. Wondering. Questioning, "Who is this Black person coming to our school...?" This was in my head. Clearly, I didn't know what they were thinking. No one yelled. No one was mean. No one said anything to me. Not one word.

For a moment, it seemed like even the birds stopped singing. I knew I needed to make it through the front door, to the office. I remember, someone, an adult—at the office—asking me if I was lost... "Yes, Ma'am," I replied. I was completely lost. More so than she could ever have known.

I found my way to my first class. Someone showed me to my homeroom. The homeroom teacher directed me to the next class. Some of the teachers were nice, some were not. They had their jobs to do. Not one student reached out. That was my day. All day. Every day.

Boy, it showed! That first report card—standing in front of my father—I had four Ds and two Cs. He knew I was a hard worker; he knew this was very difficult for me—beyond what I could manage. I recall his face and his validating, encouraging words, "Just remember, continue working hard. Want it to get better..." It didn't get any better.

That first day, lunch came around. I found the cafeteria. The room was large, lined with long tables, filled with the bustle of students, and a mass of white faces. I found the end of a table with no students. I made my way over and put my tray down. Every single one of the students got up from the table, laughed, and walked away. There I was sitting, alone, at this long table. That same day, on the school bus home, I was beaten up. That was my first day at BCC.

It did get a little better. Back then, it was common to shower after gym class and re-dress before you go back to class. I remember the teacher pulling me aside saying, "You—you won't have to take a shower." Once again, the message that I was somehow half-human was loud and clear. Who wanted this person with dark skin in the shower with white girls? Consequently, I never had to take a shower after gym.

In 11th grade, the counselor called me in for "guidance" and told me, "Because your brain..." (she actually said this) "...because your brain is smaller, I'm going to recommend that you change from academic study to commercial so you can learn to type and take shorthand." Of course, back then you did what somebody in authority told you to do. So, I switched. Then she advised, "The only office you would ever be able to work for is the Federal government. Since you live so close to Washington, DC, it would be good for you to take typing and shorthand and pass the United States Civil Service Exam; then you could get a job as a clerk or typist with the Federal government." Clearly, she thought she was helping me.

I followed her direction. I didn't even discuss it with my parents. They probably would have agreed with her; segregation was still very much a part of our lives. So, that's what I did. I graduated. I took the civil service exam and got a clerk-typist job. And hated it!

By that time, I had embraced my family's strong value—and love—for learning, school, and education. I decided to go to college. During the day I worked. At night I took classes and studied. Pretty soon I earned an undergraduate degree in education.

I share this to say that everything I experienced helped me... It helped me to know who I was. It helped me to see that there was nothing wrong with me—the system was broken. It helped me appreciate how I grew up, my family, what I had inside myself, and my connection with nature. I am so thankful for my childhood years. Carefree years of feeling safe and loved. That's what my high school experience did for me. Yes, I went through hell and I came out the other side a stronger, wiser person.

I excelled in college. I worked very hard to make up for the substandard education. After I got married, I went back to college—part-time—for a Master's Degree in Business and Public Administration. I didn't stop there... I went on and completed a Doctorate Degree in Early and Middle Childhood Education. All in all, after high school, part-time, it took me about 32 years.

That's the kind of person I am...

I give credit to my mother and father for the way they valued education and encouraged us. For the freedom we had within our home. And I also give credit to those massive, beautiful, virgin woods...

I turned the corner on education. Now the blocks in my life had to do with growing up in Black racist America—and my health.

When I got married, I was five foot nine inches and weighed 99 pounds. Genetically, my family was super-duper tall. Long and lanky.

Back then we didn't have television. Which meant our entertainment came from music or the natural world. Indoors, I fell in love with symphonic music.

Outdoors, I fell in love with nature and movement. In nature, things are always moving. Changing. Evolving. The air current stirring the leaves. The frogs hopping. The worms surfacing, creeping along after a rain. In nature nothing stands still.

Our life was changing too… Soon after we got married, I had a baby girl. I breastfed and started taking the birth control pill, a brand-new medication on the market. My weight doubled. In fact, I hit over 200 pounds.

I talked to my doctor, the same one who prescribed the birth control. He had no clue about nutrition or movement. Sadly, it's not much better today. So my doctor wrote me another prescription, this time for diet pills. Basically amphetamines. Speed. As an aside, these pills were eventually taken off the market.

I lost the weight so fast. Along with a bunch of heart muscle. Due to the side effects, diet pills were only prescribed for four to six weeks. After the prescription ended, the doctor's orders were to, "Go back to your regular lifestyle." I followed his directions. I went back to my regular habits and routines which included daily birth control pills. Not surprisingly, I gained the weight back—plus. The numbers on the scale kept creeping higher and higher. I was extremely concerned.

A trip back to the doctor harvested another round of diet pills. The weight miraculously melted away. Six weeks later the prescription ended—I quickly ballooned again. With each cycle I got heavier and heavier. At one point, I gained so much weight I could literally take my boob and throw it over the other shoulder! I felt terrible. I just did not understand what was happening to my body.

Finally, I put a stop to the diet pills. Then I tried the "grapefruit diet." The "eat half of whatever you normally eat" diet. The "starve yourself" diet. Nobody was saying anything about the birth control pills or nutrition or movement.

One day, I heard a doctor who practiced medicine in my area. Dr. Gabe Mirkin had a call-in radio show. I happened to tune in and heard him say, loud and clear, "DIETS DON'T WORK." By this point, I had been trying diets for ten years!

Dr. Mirkin said, "If you want to take better care of yourself, here's what you do: eat fruits. Vegetables. Whole grains. Beans. Seeds. Nuts. And, occasionally, a small amount of animal protein. Oh, and, you have to move."

His prescription for movement was walking—ideally daily. Enough to get your heart rate up 20 beats above your resting rate and keep it there for 30 minutes without stopping. He encouraged people to start out slow and easy. He suggested people keep a log so they could track their progress. Speed, distance, heart rate, etc. And, on the radio show, he gave us instructions about how to measure our resting heart rate.

Dr. Mirkin was a Harvard guy who also happened to be a long-distance runner. His race was the Boston marathon, along with other races of varying distances. I said to myself, "Okay, I'm going to try that..." I listened to his show every day. People would call in with all kinds of questions. He talked about health, fitness, and nutrition. That was his thing. His message was simple: "To be healthy... you gotta be fit. And you gotta eat right." Boy, I heard him loud and clear!

I started preparing meals accordingly. Fruits, vegetables, whole grains, beans, seeds, and nuts. My family adjusted to the new lifestyle (they had to!).

At some point, I decided to go beyond Dr. Mirkin's suggestions. First, I stopped eating red meat. Then I stopped the poultry. Over time, I stopped eating seafood. I checked in with my doctor to make sure I was in good health and not deficient in anything. It didn't take long before I began looking and feeling better, and my body started shedding the excess weight.

I started this journey in 1969. Over the years, these changes have become a foundational part of the lifestyle I embrace today.

Of course, since the 1960s, science has made many new discoveries about how to take better care of our health and fitness. As I read the research, I began to notice that scientists were looking at the natural world and learning a lot from nature. I was curious. I knew I was on a solid path to better health and nutrition. However, it wasn't enough. A part of me—probably because I was feeling so good—wanted to learn more. I wanted to take what I was doing, learning, and experiencing to another level. So, I started looking beyond Dr. Mirkin's work.

Through the literature, a framework for my lifestyle began to emerge. A framework which I now call: *Nature's System-based Lifestyle Training Program*. This program is grounded in natural systems. The systems we find in nature where the woods, the trees, varieties of animals, flora and fauna, insects, and birds are all vital parts of a whole system. Systems intricately interconnected with the sun, the sky, the soil, and the seasons. Interdependent—supporting one another. Nature and nature's wisdom has become the focal point for my life and my training program.

In nature, there is a balance between passion and perseverance. I learned that from childhood, I just didn't realize it back then. Think about it... it took a balance of passion and perseverance to carve out the canyons, the glaciers, the cliffs, and the lowlands. Plus, deep down, I knew that if I was going to hold on to my healthy lifestyle, I would need both. I would need passion for my system as a whole and perseverance to keep going.

So, I coined the word *passionverance*.

Passionverance is holistic. It considers the entire human system. Passionverance is about living your entire life naturally, guided by the greatest natural system—Mother Nature.

In my experience, you can't have true health unless you have both. Passion and perseverance go hand-in-hand. For instance, if I eat the wrong things, I can't do the running I want to do. If I run without the proper nutrition, I'll get injured. If I get injured, I can't run. If I can't run, my mind and body don't feel so great. Can you see how one reinforces and supports the other?

For the training program I developed principles—a matrix, if you like... If you are going to make any change in your life, you must have internal strength, strength inside your body and brain, or nothing will change.

The interplay between mind and body is another principal nature helps us see.... Change won't last unless both the mind and body are interacting and reinforcing each other. For example, I can be running (physical body) along quite happily, when I see a hill in the distance. I know my legs, heart, and lungs can get me up that hill. But what about my mind? I know my mind has the power to get me up that hill or stall me before I even start. If I approach that hill with positive thinking (the mind) and start saying to myself, "Oh good, there's a great hill. This is a good opportunity to test out my hill training,"—all is well. If, on the other hand, I allow my thoughts (the mind) to think, "Geez, that's a big hill, there's no way I can run up that," then I will end up walking (the body) and feeling defeated (emotions).

On reflection, I think this is one thing attending that integrated school taught me. I knew, without a doubt, I had undying internal—mind/body—strength. To survive I had to be strong, passionate about learning, and determined to succeed.

The next thing in nature's principles is nutrition and movement. When in harmony, nutrition and movement are a powerful team. Influencing and reinforcing each other. If you want sustainable change, you can't use diet alone—some kind of movement is vital.

When your mind and body are working together and your nutrition and movement are in sync, at some point you will reach—and cross—the lifestyle change line. What does this mean? Well, whatever you have given up—junk food, processed food, sweets, candy, whatever—Mother Nature, through your body, kicks in extra support to help you maintain the change. How? Well, once you have been eating fruits, veggies, whole grains, beans, seeds, and nuts for a while and someone takes you out for your birthday or dinner or whatever, and you eat something that you haven't eaten in a long time, you will not feel good. Your body will rebel with signals like nausea, diarrhea, and lethargy. This is natural. This is the body telling you, "I don't like this. I'm not happy. Let's not do this again."

You see, our bodies have a wisdom. Our bodies are smarter than the doctors. Our bodies are definitely smarter than our thoughts. Once your system (body/mind) crosses this natural line, all you have to do is listen closely to your body. Your body will tell you exactly what you need—and what you don't need.

Trust me, there are multi-billion dollar fast and processed food industries working hard to pull you back over the line—the wrong way. This isn't easy. I still have ongoing challenges, and so will you. My mother made this incredible banana pudding that I loved growing up. When I would go home, I'd get some pressure—especially from my siblings, "Oh, come on, Betty. You're going to make Mother feel bad. She spent extra time—especially for you." I'd have to explain, "I appreciate it, but I don't eat that anymore." Once you cross the line, challenges will come your way too. If you can hold on, or hold off, you will be rewarded.

This brings me to nature's final principle—healthier outcomes for the rest of your life.

I'm 81 years old. I take no medication. Not even over-the-counter stuff. I don't get headaches. I don't get stomach problems. I don't get sick. Not even a common cold.

My immune system is so balanced because of my nutrition and the movement. It's not that I haven't been exposed to sickness. Over my career, I did a lot of work on Indian reservations and remote villages in Alaska. So remote that one time I flew into Anchorage, and then had another three-hour plane ride in a little four-seater puddle jumper to get to these villages. Once there, the villages would be rampant with tuberculosis (TB), dysentery, other bacteria, and viruses. I never got sick. My colleagues did, but not me…

Remember, our immune systems are a part of nature's wisdom. If your immune system is out of balance, for example, it doesn't turn off after fighting off germs, viruses, even stress. It will react with an inflammatory response, which could lead to cancer cell growth. That's natural. A sign. Of course, science now knows that an overactive immune system—one that's constantly on—causes all sorts of problems in the body: cancer, autoimmune disorders, gut issues, anxiety, etc.

Nature also pursues excellence. Take the Grand Canyon, for example—one of the wonders of the world. People come from all over to visit, hike, and take in its magnificence. The Grand Canyon surpasses human expectations. Made drip by drip over eons. Patience. One of nature's principles is patience. We can learn from nature. Model her speed and pace.

Me? I have learned patience. Every morning, I cut and peel ginger and turmeric. I make a tea, along with cumin seed and distilled water. I take the time to steep the tea in a teapot. Why distilled water? Well, I did an experiment with a philodendron plant. I rooted two. One in a jar with city (tap) water. The other in a jar with distilled water. Both plants were both exposed to the same heat and light. I let the water evaporate. Once the water was gone, what did I find? The jar with the distilled water was completely clear. The jar with the tap water was coated with a white powdery residue. I have no idea what that powder was, however, I do know I don't want that stuff inside my body.

So, distilled water goes into my teapot. I take my time. I feel the roots. Then I smell the roots. I absorb the texture. Then I steep the tea. As the tea steeps, the roots change. The smell changes. The texture changes. The whole process from start to finish is wonderfully meditative. As, I believe, nature intended.

The final principle in *Nature's System-based Lifestyle Training Program* is harnessing nature's ability to repair. Years ago, I realized I needed to learn and unlearn some things. For example, I had to learn that diets don't work. Yes, you might shed some weight quickly, however, over a lifetime it's not sustainable. I had to learn how and what my body needed to restore and maintain optimal health. This for me includes balance, strength, and good health.

Remember, you, me, we—are all a part of nature. That's a foundational principle.

I had to learn how to structure my day-to-day life more effectively. Slowly. Over time. I learned how to eat, prepare food, shop differently. It was the same for movement. I learned that I needed to get out and move every day. I experimented and adjusted my day accordingly. Gradually. Over time. Remember, I was 29 years old when I started this journey. Now, I am 81 and still running 80-plus miles a week.

Nature takes her time. Change is a process. It takes time—another of nature's core principles.

I also had to learn how to listen to my body from head to toe. I learned to tune in, listen, sense what my body is doing. What it is taking in. What my body is telling me. What it needs. If I have a stomachache, I figure it out. I check inside, "Hey, what's going on, why is my stomach feeling off?" Honestly, since I have been on fruits, vegetables, whole grains, beans, seeds, and nuts, I don't get stomach issues anymore. I have learned to notice, and focus on, what *is* working.

And I learned that another principle was planning. Walking turned into running marathons, ultra-marathons, and 6-day races. Over the years, I have completed marathons all over the world. I have run a marathon on every continent, with the exception of China, where I ran The Great Wall Half Marathon.

Of course, I knew I would be away from home. In order to stay well, I had to plan ahead. I prepped—as much as possible—so I could eat what I would normally. As a long-distance runner the right kind of protein is vital. I packed the food I needed—mostly a suitcase full of chickpeas and chia seeds.

As I mentioned earlier, my job took me all over the United States. I remember going to a restaurant with a colleague in Montana. It was a steak place. My friend was a steak person. I don't make judgements about what other people choose to eat. We arrived later in the evening. There was not much on the menu for me, so I asked the server for some wheat toast. "We don't serve wheat toast," he said. "But we do have wheat toast with our bacon, lettuce, cheese and tomato sandwich. Would you like that?" he offered. I said, "Okay, how about giving me a bacon, lettuce, cheese, and tomato sandwich. Hold the bacon. Hold the cheese. Hold the tomato. No mayonnaise. Just the lettuce and the toast, please." He said, "Okay, we can do that, but I'll have to charge you for the full sandwich." "That's fine," I said. It was late at night. We're in Montana in a small town. I didn't plan ahead.

In 1989, I ran my second marathon in Moscow, Russia. Wow! So much to see there... However, food-wise, not so much. The city didn't seem to accommodate much of anything except boiled potatoes and sliced tomatoes. Consequently, I ate boiled potatoes and tomatoes for breakfast, lunch, and dinner—for two weeks. Tip: plan ahead.

Over the years, I have learned how to navigate restaurants, parties, holidays, friends, and family. I simply bring my food. I explain to the wait staff that I am on a special diet. I hang out, eat my food, and enjoy my friends just like everyone else.

The final principle here is—no excuses! I plan ahead. I say no. I stay on track. No excuses. Harnessing the wisdom of nature has taken me from a 200-plus pounds, smoking, sitting on the sofa, eating bon bons woman—to a fit, active, healthy 81-year-old. I shovel snow, I rake leaves, and I do my own yard work.

Recently, I was up in a cedar tree with a saw trimming branches. I was literally in the tree surrounded by the essence of cedar, the feel of the soft wood, the warm sunshine. It was so beautiful. My next-door neighbor heard branches falling; he comes around and says, "Hey Ms. Betty! What are you doing up there?" "Trimming my tree," I reply. He offers to help—waving his chainsaw. I, of course, thanked him and said, "No, thank you... I am quite happy moving and using my body; sawing back and forth." The activity uses my muscles—from my back to my arms, and all the way down my sides. Plus, I'm outside in the fresh air, with the sunshine, surrounded by this beautiful cedar tree. Needless to say, since then they've left me alone.

Nature has helped me learn how to move the barriers out of my way. I came to grips with being Black in America. I can't change America. I can't erase segregation—wish I could, but I can't. I need to do what I can do to live the best life I can... I know that I will, intentionally or unintentionally, always run into some level of discrimination. I have learned to handle that. The looks. The comments. The snubs. I live my life in spite of that.

I am thankful to have found a different way of living. An alternative to the lifestyle that is so prevalent here in the United States. I have seen through the barrage of messages which encourage convenience food, poor nutrition, and minimal movement.

Today, of course, we have the research to support that eating whole foods, nuts, and grains combined with daily movement—things that the natural world already provides for us—are key factors in good health and longevity. In fact, the research is beginning to support that our lifestyle choices have a powerful influence on preventing conditions such as obesity, diabetes, and heart attacks—more so than our genetic profiles. This is great news: just because your mother or father had X genes, we know that this is no longer a recipe for disaster. Today, with more access to functional medicine and holistic health and healing practices, people have options—the choice—to try alternative paths. With the help and guidance of nature and the natural world, we can do a lot to live long, healthy lives.

I am living proof. I still run ultra-marathons. I run in minimal shoes: Vivo barefoot shoes which support the natural use of my feet. Flat with a penetration proof sole, the shoes are designed with a wide toe box and no arch support, this allows my feet to do what nature intended them to do. According to my podiatrist, my feet and legs have only got stronger!

Here is a funny story. The shoe company invited me to New York to meet *Born to Run* author/ultra-runner Christopher McDougal. I honestly didn't know about him... We both arrived early. We sat on the floor, in the store, chatting. He told me about Tarahumara Indians from the Copper Canyon region of Mexico. He described all the issues he had with recurring plantar fasciitis and his journey to minimal shoes—and, I might add—no more plantar fasciitis. Then, he told me about how the Tarahumara ran 200 to 300 miles on chia seed.

Of course, I was fascinated and very curious about chia seed. Later, I bought some organic chia seed and started trying it—gradually—using nature's measured process. To my surprise, I found that I could run—seemingly forever. I was blossoming into an ultra-ultra-runner. My body needed to run longer, organized, timed races. I found all sorts of races from 24, 48, 72 hours—all the way up to six days. I fact, last year, I completed a six-day race. I ran six days and six nights with little break in minimal shoes.

These courses are generally designed in loops of three miles or so. Usually the longer the race, the shorter the loop. I plan ahead. I bring all the food I normally eat. I set-up my little table with distilled water. If the race has refrigeration, then I bring the patties I make which contain protein, complex carbohydrates, polyunsaturated fat, usually olive oil—frozen—on the airplane in my checked luggage. Then they go into the hotel's freezer. This ensures that I will have the protein (chickpeas, beans, chia seed) and the carbohydrates (nuts, seeds, grains) my body needs.

Chia seed is truly a gift of nature. Those tiny seeds are packed full of so many vitamins and minerals and protein! Plus, they last on my kitchen counter for six months. Chia seed is a big part of what I eat and/or drink during the six-day races.

I use a log with the day and time listed on one side, my food items listed on the other side, and reminders about changing my shoes. And I foam roll my muscles every 24 hours—I add that to the log too. Other runners don't take the time. I do... One of nature's principles: take time. I have never had to go into the medical tent in any of these ultra runs.

Johns Hopkins University has been doing research on aging and energy financed by the National

Institutes of Health. Researchers have been monitoring my running, my aging, and my energy for years. I am too much of an outlier for the group due to age and fitness levels. I am proud to be the exception.

My running cadence is timed with a metronome. A drumbeat metronome. My body is attuned to this beat of the drum. It's completely natural. I don't have to think about it. My body just responds. I waste no energy. Just like nature.

So that's my life. Living by nature's principles… What else?

I have to tell you this story… We moved into this house which backs on to Rock Creek Park with virgin woods. I didn't realize what I was doing at the time, but after some years I figured it out. I was letting nature in. How? Well, it's an older house. The first thing I did was remove the internal walls. Now the house is more open. Then gradually, over time, I added skylights in the kitchen, living room, bedroom, and the office. At the back of the house, we took out the solid walls and added all glass.

Now, I see the woods, the trees, and the sky all day long. I have a reading chair which swings. I can do a 360-degree turn to look at my woods anytime I want…

I like to do puzzles. Right now, I am working on Shavonne's Blue Vase. I still work coaching walkers and runners, plus I teach deep water running for the county government.

Over the last 50 years or so I have run more than a hundred thousand miles. How do I know? Well, some years ago *Runner's World* did the calculation. Years later, the magazine published an article on aging and running, and they profiled me as an ageless runner.

I have two teenage grandsons who live close by. Over the years, we have spent a lot of time together, and nature has been a big part of their lives too. I remember a funny story. A family of wasps set up their home near my front door. My grandsons, maybe three and four years old at the time, and I made friends with them. We developed a language. A wasp language. We talked to them. We sang to them. We would sit in chairs right below the nest— they never bothered us. However, one day our neighbors came to visit and they sat in the very same chairs, and they got stung! Yikes!

Nevertheless, the boys were convinced that Mother Nature is good, and those wasps were our special friends. They got to the point where they would not even step on an ant. "Watch out! That's somebody's mother," they would shout.

Currently, my grandsons are helping me train for another six-day race. They run with me every day for an hour. Watching my grandsons grow into fine young men with a strong connection to the natural world is such a gift. I am so proud.

Here is a fun fact: the University of Norway Department of Science and Technology has been developing a way to measure fitness age versus chronological age. My fitness age is 32 years old. My resting heart rate is 29 to 32 beats a minute. I have an annual check-up with my doctors. They are all absolutely amazed.

What's my daily routine? The first thing I do is wake up my joints. I start with my ankles, circling them. Then I move up the body: knees, hips, neck, arms, elbows. Then I go into muscle strengthening, which is a combination of planks, plank holds, resistance band training, flexibility, and balance work. In the background I have nature, the sound of water and, of course, a view of the woods.

I finish with Tai Chi. This is my 35th year of practice. The Tai Chi pulls it all together: strengthening, flexibility, balance, relaxation. Then I sit quietly for a few minutes, listening to the water, the soft music, the sounds. Sometimes my mind floats. Sometimes it's just there—noticing. I see the trees, the birds, the insects—right now we have a lot of cicadas. Then I am ready for the day.

I have a great life... There is no doubt in my mind that I owe that to Mother Nature. I learned to respect her wisdom and found so many ways through—food, movement, sights, sounds—to add her wisdom into my entire life. Mind. Body. Spirit. Surroundings.

Through nature, I have learned to live in the moment and learned to let go of things I cannot control. Nature is my coach and my guide; with the running and the eating, it all works together. I take what I learn from the natural world and put it back into my body.

In short, I see myself as a part of nature. I live my life according to nature's principles. The truth is that we are all part of the natural world. We can't forget that...

———

# MOVEMENT MATTERS

*"If you rest, you rust."*
                           – Helen Hayes

**I LOVE THIS QUOTE...** It brings back fond memories of a colleague who was working on recovering from a life of inactivity. After a knee replacement, she became even more determined to get into shape. We were accountability buddies. At the end of the day, I would show up at her desk, "You ready?" I would ask. "Yep" she would say, "you know, when you rest, you rust." I would smile, "Darn right," I would reply, "Let's do this...". Then we would lace up and head out on the trail together. Those words became our mantra and held a truth—about the importance of movement for a healthy mind and body. A truth I still abide by today. Thank you, Nancy!

Within these incredible stories you will notice two consistent themes: movement and nature. We'll get to the *Why Nature?* chapter in a bit. First, I want to dive into the question, "Why is movement so important in the healing and recovery process?"

When I am helping someone who is actively working on integrating—shifting—their grief, loss, or trauma story, part of the work is to begin to embrace what I call the *Cornerstones of Health:*

- Quality sleep
- Water—lots of it
- Natural, nutritious food
- Breath work/mindfulness
- Time in nature
- Mindset
- Movement

Let me be clear... I prefer using the word "movement" over "exercise." I appreciate these are two sides of the same coin and language is important. If I power through the *Cornerstones of Health* with someone who has been sedentary for a while or has an aversion to the "E" word (some people do...) or someone who feels impossibly out of shape or depressed, I will get several reactions: the eyes glaze, the body stiffens, resistance settles in. The word "movement" is softer, gentler, more expansive, natural. After all, it's undeniable, that on some level, we humans do move—right?

Then, once we begin to connect movement with time in nature, a powerful synergy begins to stir. It's a wonderful process to witness. A particular memory comes to mind. Several years ago, I was working with a woman (I'll call her Pam) who lost her son to suicide. Her world, and life, as she knew it screeched to a halt. Completely shattered. Devastated. Unbearable pain. After about a year (the first year is often the hardest), the spring came. Slowly Pam began to warm to the idea of sitting in a sunny window for a few minutes—just noticing the changes. The hues shifting, the new growth, the bird activity. She loved birds—something, in the deep grief, she had forgotten about. Pam bought a bird feeder and placed it strategically outside her window. More birds came: all shapes and sizes and colors. More glimmers of joy began to surface, a moment at a time. With the promise of new life and brighter, warmer days, it was like something began unfurling within Pam too. Soon Pam ventured outside. Refilling the bird seed. Moving her body as she ambled around, noticing her garden. Then, one day Pam took a walk through the neighborhood. Then a bit further, to a local park with water and trees and baby geese. Her family celebrated Easter, a spring birthday, and a beloved sibling came to visit. As the spring advanced, Pam began noticing, moving, and feeling life again.

When it comes to our emotional wounds, our traumas, anything from a car wreck to the loss of a loved one to violence, abuse, and neglect—movement plays a vital role in the healing process. Trauma is stored in the brain (the nervous system) and the physical body (the tissue, muscles, fascia). Physical movement begins to open the lines of communication between the body and the brain. Connecting the dots. Putting the puzzle pieces together. Movement helps our nervous systems restore balance by burning off stress and tension held in the body and, at the same time, important "feel good" endorphins are released.

Cardiovascular movement is particularly helpful because it stimulates biochemical changes in the brain by increasing oxygen, enhancing blood flow, and encouraging neuroplasticity. And, because it's a two-way street—mind/body-body/mind—regular, intentional movement helps remove the build-up of toxins created by stress, tension, fear, anxiety, etc. In time, our brain, nervous system, and other vital organs begin to feel more settled. Grounded. We might notice our mood begin to shift. Once this happens, then, again slowly, we may start to see our world—and life—from a different perspective.

Both personally and professionally, I have witnessed the power of the synergy that is created between movement, the natural world, and healing. Everything from simply feeling "a bit better" to, as in my case, feeling like layers of grief and loss have been shed.

Thanks to advances in science and technology, we now have data that helps us understand why movement coupled with time in nature is so important. Studies have shown that activities such as walking, running, hiking, and biking can help ease symptoms related to anxiety, depression, post-traumatic stress disorder, high blood pressure, diabetes, etc. In her book *Dopamine Nation*—which I highly recommend—Dr. Anna Lembke, Chief of the Stanford Addiction Medicine Dual Diagnosis Clinic, eloquently writes about the power and the why of exercise:

*"Exercise increases many of the neurotransmitters involved in positive mood regulation: dopamine, serotonin, norepinephrine, epinephrine, endocannabinoids, and endogenous opioid peptides (endorphins). Exercise contributes to the birth of new neurons and supporting glial cells."*

To be clear, you don't have to be some athletic super-human to reap these benefits. Dr. Lembke concludes:

*"A key to well-being is for us to get off the couch and move our real bodies. I tell my patients, just walking in your neighborhood for 30 minutes a day can make a difference. The evidence is indisputable: exercise [movement] has a more profound effect and sustained positive effect on mood, anxiety, cognition, energy, and sleep than any pill I can prescribe."*

That is a powerful statement...

———

# MINDSET:
## LEMONS TO LEMONADE

*"Someone I once loved gave me a box full of darkness. It took me years to understand that this, too, was a gift."*

– Mary Oliver

IF YOU IMAGINE a house, think about mindset as the foundation. Mindsets are formed by a mixture of experiences: education (formal and informal), culture (social, religious, political), environment (family, friends, teams, etc.). Mindsets are developed, built, and crafted over time. Mindsets support our thoughts, beliefs, and attitudes (think walls of the house). These thoughts, beliefs, and attitudes stimulate/cause our actions, choices, and behaviors (think roof of the house).

The good news is that mindsets are not fixed: they can and do change—sometimes quickly, sometimes slowly, depending on the event or situation at hand. Also, because the way mindsets are formed—partly from a collection of beliefs—they are often quite unconscious. Hidden. Out of thought awareness.

One of the struggles I have with today's pop culture and the "Seven Simple Steps to Change Your

Mindset" type of message is that changing our mindset is neither simple nor easy. As humans, with a lovely frontal cortex, we have the ability to think consciously, to reflect; even have opposing thoughts. Here's the rub: at the same time, we are often oblivious to the underlying beliefs which are driving those thoughts.

Here's the chain of command: thoughts lead to memories—visual and body sensations—which lead to, or spark, deeper, often unconscious beliefs. Plus, this nervous system domino effect happens in a nano-second. To varying extents, this is true for most of us 95 percent of the time.

Working with people in my practice, uncovering those unconscious beliefs and making them conscious, is an important part of the healing process. When we bring an unconscious belief into the light—the process of change and shifting that belief—can begin. Once the belief shifts, then our energy, attitude, perspective—mindset—also begins to shift. This is powerful because it presents an opportunity or the space to consciously choose to do, or see, something different.

Take a moment to reflect. Check in. What have we covered so far?

- Mindsets are a natural part of being human.
- Mindsets are formed from messages: environmental, cultural, family, media, sports—you name it!

- Mindsets are deep and complex—often unconscious.
- Mindsets and beliefs have a direct influence on each other.
- Mindsets can, and do, change— sometimes very quickly.

As you reflect, what beliefs might be limiting you? Again, we *all* have them. The work is to discover our unhelpful beliefs and shift them toward something more beneficial.

Some of the limiting beliefs I held were deeper and more complex. Childhood stuff. Unhelpful beliefs that lurked in the dark corners of my mind, holding me back, that—over the years—with the assistance of some wonderful therapists, I have managed to work through, exchanging them for more constructive content. I do encourage the assistance of a well-trained professional when embarking on this work—particularly if you are digging into deeper issues. That said, it is possible to cut through some of the "easier" limiting beliefs by yourself (practical steps to follow).

## Stories and beliefs

As humans we are incredibly gifted. Nature (or whatever you believe) has provided us with a frontal cortex—a vast, intricate, awe-inspiring super-computer—housed within a nervous system that we cannot even begin to understand and fully appreciate. No other creature on the planet has the ability to create stories, beliefs, or movies, that hum along gently in the background, complete with technicolor, narration, and surround sound.

How are our beliefs, the stories we tell ourselves, created? In part—a big part—from tiny whisps of seeds that were planted way back when. Of course, just like the dandelion, not every seed will sprout. Grow. Take hold. Some will. Some won't. Why? We are not sure; neuroscientists are working hard to figure this out.

To illustrate, consider… How often are you going about your day—everything is fine—when something unforeseen interrupts the version of your movie? Generally, it's some sort of external event. Traffic. Kids. Partner. Boss. Money. This disruption (event) causes a cascade of internal changes. Shifts in thinking, "Ugh! Why does everything go wrong?" Shifts in mood: sour, grumpy, irritable. Shifts in the body: tightness, tension, clenching (jaw, stomach, hands). And shifts in behavior: sighing, slamming, blaming. This process takes place within our nervous system at lightning speed. What is one of the components that triggers our nervous systems to react/respond in this way? Our personal beliefs.

When we feel stuck, overwhelmed, anxious and/or we have a sense that we are overreacting to a thing or an event, this is often a sign that a core belief has been activated. Sometimes, this reaction is helpful—even protective.

Here's a real-life example: imagine I'm hiking over a sandstone outcropping on a warm, summer afternoon. My buddy steps to the edge to soak in the epic view, almost stepping on a big, fat, copperhead peacefully curled up basking in the sun. Of course, she (my buddy, not the snake…) jumps back, a little shaken, keeping a respectful distance. Curious, I take a peek too. We leave the snake in peace, basking in its glory. Later, maybe a mile down the trail, something else quickly slithers across our path. Yikes! Instinctively, we jump out of our skins and move swiftly down the trail. From that point, my brain is on high alert, keen to spot more of our silent, slithery friends before they see us. This is an example of a protective, survival-type reaction. Interestingly, many scientists believe that our fear response to snakes and spiders is deeply wired into our DNA.

It's a bit different when a seed belief gets triggered. How do we know? What is the difference? Let's go back to our everyday events: traffic, kids, partners, bosses, money, and running late examples.

Running or being late for things is a common, uniquely human experience. How do you respond when you are running late? Frustration? Stressed with increased heart rate and heat in the body? Anger? Yelling at any poor sap who happens to get in your way? Maybe you are the quiet type, cool as a cucumber on the outside, yet silently smoldering on the inside? Take a moment to note your particular brand of reaction (story/belief).

Now step back a bit, away from your reaction. Imagine the same running late event with three different humans—people who are not you. As if you are simply a casual observer or a fly on the wall. I do this in session a lot. It's fun. Let's play this out: same event, three different people, and you as a casual observer. How might, or could, they see, respond, think about running late? What are some other or alternate stories people could tell themselves about the running late event? Take a moment and come up with three different responses/stories. Then, we'll work through some options together:

> Person A response: _____
> Person B response: _____
> Person C response: _____

Okay! Great. Let's break it down. I will add my ideas and highlight some possible beliefs:

Person A: As soon as she realizes she's running late, she makes a call to let whoever is waiting know the situation. She is operating on the belief/story that, "I'm okay. People will understand."

Person B: Berates himself all day, "I was so late this morning, I hate being late." The belief/story, "I'm a bad person," has been triggered.

Person C: Takes a few breaths while reminding herself that, "It is fine, I'm fine, and it will be fine." This triggers the story/belief, "There's no real threat here," and the feeling, "I'm okay."

Evidently, Person C has been working hard in therapy... Joking aside, hopefully you are beginning to see that we have all learned to respond to everyday life events in a myriad of ways and that many of our responses arise from stories we have learned, and in turn, those stories, over time, have crystalized into beliefs. These beliefs lay down roots deep in our nervous systems and become *the* "truth." We see this all the time in politics, religion, conflict, social divide—it's that "I'm right, he/she is wrong" type of mindset.

From the above example, I am hoping that you are beginning to see a couple of things:

- That being late is, in truth, simply an event. A uniquely human event. Let's face it: dogs, cats, and horses don't react to "being late."
- Being late (an event) means different things to different people. Based on cultural norms and other stories we have absorbed about "being late," we have created distinct beliefs and our nervous systems have, over time, learned to respond accordingly.
- With awareness we can begin to shift unhelpful stories and beliefs that limit us—

keeping us stuck—and work toward creating more helpful, preferred perspectives: stories which, with time, practice, and patience, will become new beliefs to better serve us in our present-day lives.

## Seed and core beliefs

It's important to recognize that we have two types of beliefs:

- Seed beliefs: beliefs we have learned along the way.
- Core beliefs: deeply wired survival reactions (snakes, spiders, heights, etc.).

Clearly, there is power behind both types of beliefs. Core (survival) beliefs tend to be housed much more deeply out of conscious awareness. Seed beliefs tend to live a little closer to the surface. However, both seed and core beliefs are directly connected to mindset—how we see the world, the stories we tell ourselves, what we think, and how we respond. Harnessing and understanding the power of our mindset gives us the ability to make lemonade out of lemons.

As mentioned, another intriguing thing about mindsets is that they can—and do—change.

Because so much of our day-to-day human operations is going on under the hood—out of conscious awareness—catching, naming, and reframing an unhelpful or unskillful belief can be tricky. The following is a personal example adapted from the first book in this series *Never Too Late: Inspiration, Motivation, and Sage Advice from 7 Later-In-Life Athletes.*

*...We grow up and head out into the world. We make all sorts of smart, logical, front-brain decisions. Yet, we are also very capable of making decisions that are not so helpful. If it were simply our thoughts running the show, I contend that we would be much better at using that highly logical thinking part of our brain, which—logically (again, pun intended)—would lead to super logical—helpful behavior.*

*If it were that easy, wouldn't we all have our gym bags neatly packed by the door ready for the chime of that early morning alarm bell? Wouldn't it be effortless to spring out of bed just because our thoughts commanded it? Wouldn't we all be fit and healthy simply because we "know" it's good for us? I can tell you, at least in my experience, this is generally not the case.*

*The point I am trying to make is that somewhere along the way we have all soaked up beliefs that are unhelpful. Beliefs that limit us. In doing my own work around the topic of motivation I realized that I had a sneaky limiting belief around "being lazy". Once I was able to put this deeper sense, or feeling, into words I was able to work with it.*

*When I fact-check my 58-year-old self I am*

*clearly not lazy. I run, hike, write, own and operate a small business, and take care of a family and a home. That "belief" was clearly old seed stuff coming up. Also, I know no one comes out of the chute thinking/believing "I'm lazy." Right then, I knew this was an unhelpful seed belief vs. a core belief—which interestingly provided some relief. OK, I thought, "I'm not inherently lazy; that's unhelpful seed stuff. I can change that. Cool!"*

*With a bit more digging I was able to trace the origins of this unhelpful belief to my early teens. Somewhere, during that glorious period when I was sleeping until noon, obnoxious, and expected the world to revolve around me—I connected with the sense of soaking up seed messages from my environment with a "you're so lazy" theme. The originating sources were likely my family—around chores (particularly cleaning my room), and the school system—stuff around "not trying hard enough"—which I, in my adolescent brain, internalized as "I'm lazy." That's the best I could come up with.*

Yes, that seed was likely planted over 40 years ago. One important thing to know about our beliefs is that they don't adhere to a time zone. Days. Weeks. Years. That's not how they roll. Our seed beliefs are more like weather patterns. Or the sky. It's there. We take it for granted and don't think about it too much—until we look out of the window and see storm clouds when we had grand plans to go to the pool.

When a seed belief gets activated, we can notice it in a variety of ways: thoughts, feelings, physical sensations, images (mind movies), sometimes even sounds. My "I'm lazy" seed belief generally presented itself as a thought, actually more accurately, as a little voice that appears to come out of nowhere from somewhere near the back of my head. That "voice," very quickly, led to a feeling and corresponding body sensation. The feeling: defeated. The body sensation: heavy. For me, this was often followed by a flood of more unhelpful thoughts (misery loves company...) that kept validating all the reasons I should not lace up and go for that run.

I affectionately refer to our unhelpful or limiting seed beliefs as gifts that keep on giving.

Please know, we *all* have helpful and unhelpful beliefs. It's part of being human. The problem with the unhelpful ones is that they limit us. Keeping us stuck in crappy situations—jobs, relationships, finances, etc. Unhelpful beliefs are often at the core of the habits we don't like—and can't seem to kick. They drive our internal dialogue—our mental chatter: our "not good enough(s)," our "should(s)," our "I can't(s)."

When I am working with people, like a detective, I am looking for clues, the tell-tale signs of unhelpful seed beliefs. Again, once we really begin to drill down into the root, our limiting seed beliefs land in three buckets:

- Defectiveness—unworthy, not good enough, etc.
- Control—helpless, powerless, etc.
- Safety—afraid, not safe, something bad will happen, etc.

When someone uncovers or connects with a deeply-seeded unhelpful belief, their whole nervous system will respond. Feelings often flood in, along with memories (mental movies about specific events from the past), body sensations (often in the stomach, chest, throat, and eyes), and thoughts (a lot of thinking). Just like seeds, our limiting beliefs come in all shapes, sizes, and varieties.

## Uncovering seed beliefs

Imagine a sweet pea vine—soft, delicate, unruly. Yet, with time, effort, and gentle tending, I contend that our seed beliefs are totally trainable. In short, once you start to notice, uncover, and connect with a seed belief, you can begin to work with it. The work starts with two things: questions and noticing.

Questions lead to noticing and noticing leads to more questions. They are connected. It doesn't matter which one you start with. The exercise below starts with questions. Generally, questions are an effective way to open the necessary pathways in our brain, which, like a trail of breadcrumbs, will lead us to a limiting belief. Again, it is possible to do this work solo. As I said above, a well-trained coach or therapist can be immensely helpful. The first goal here is to access the system.

## Questions...

Let's get started. You will need some quiet time with a pen and paper handy. Take a couple of breaths. I will provide examples along the way...

## Step 1: Consider

As you consider the following questions, think about the past two weeks—no over thinking here—and respond to one of the questions below with short, simple statements:

- Where do I feel most stuck? (relationships, job, finances, health, etc.)

or

- What has caused me the most distress in the past two weeks? (person, place, event, behavior, etc.)

or

- Currently, what am I most dissatisfied with?

Example: Statement: *Where do I feel most stuck?* Answer: *My health*

**Step 2: Thoughts**

What are all the thoughts related to your answer in Step 1? List as many as you can, whether they make sense or not.

Example: *My thoughts related to "My health," the area I feel most stuck.*

Thought: *I feel like an old lady.*

Thought: *This discomfort in my hip is slowing down my training.*

Thought: *It will never get better.*

**Step 3: Review**

Now review your responses and see if you can identify any unhelpful beliefs.

- What stories/beliefs/themes are unhelpful? Make a note...

    *Note:* An unhelpful belief is something (a story) that hinders you. It doesn't currently serve you. It's likely untrue, generally negative, and it doesn't make sense in the context of your life today.

Example: *My unhelpful belief was "It will never get better".*

**Step 4: Notice**

Now it's time to notice, get curious, and interested, as if you are observing this process casually, like a bystander. I call this "dropping into the body." Get out of the thinking brain and connect with the body brain. Reread your statement/s. Stack your answers about the event and the corresponding belief and notice, "What is the information in your body, gut, nervous system showing/telling you?" Notice things like heat/cool, tension/openness, images, stories attached to images, language, emotions, etc. There is no right, wrong, or judgement here. As you do this, here are some questions to ask yourself:

- Where did this belief come from?
- What is this belief about?
- When did I first hear/learn about this belief?
- How old was I?
- Where was I?
- How *was* this belief helpful?
- Does this belief serve me in my current life?
  *Note:* You might not have answers to all these questions—that's okay. Also, again, no judgement. No blame. Just gentle curiosity.

Example: *The hip pain will never get better. I notice tension and anxiety swirling in my stomach and some general heat in the body.*

## Step 5: Discover

Now it's time to use what you are learning to discover. To boil it all down to form one simple "I" statement. It looks something like this, "When I look at the information from the questions (above), when

X situation happens, my thinking tells me
_____. My body shows me _____.
When I feel like this, I believe I am _____
(limiting belief).

Use the grid below to help identify some
common categories our limiting beliefs tend to fall
in. Your belief may be different. That's okay. Go
with what comes up...

| Defective | Control | Fear |
|---|---|---|
| Never good enough | Powerless | Unsafe |
| Too old/young/dumb, etc. | Never right/ always wrong | Can't trust/ rejection |
| Failure/worthless/hopeless | Not in control | Unlovable |

My example: *When I tweaked my hip, my
thinking told me, "I will never get better." My body
showed me tension, anxiety, fear. My limiting belief
was, "I am powerless."*

**Step 6: Evaluate**

Take a long hard look at your *"I am_____"*
limiting belief and ask yourself:

- Does this belief match with the facts and
  reality of my life today? Simply a yes or no
  answer.
- What would my life be like without this
  belief? List what comes to mind.
- How would I be if I didn't hold this belief?
  Imagine the ways *you* would be different.

*Note:* This is a purely logical, linear front-brain, here and now activity. Put any emotion, critical voice, or judgement aside. This is where the magic happens—you are moving unconscious back-brain stuff into front-brain consciousness. Great work!

Example: My answers:

- No. "I am powerless" does not match the facts of my life today.
- I wouldn't feel so anxious, consumed, and worried about this hip pain.
- I would remember the body heals. I would feel more confident. I have a great massage therapist who is amazing. I have been through this before. There are things I can do. I will be fine.

## Step 7: Cultivate

I love this word! What does *cultivate* mean? According to Miriam-Webster.com *cultivate* means two things:

- To prepare and use
- To foster growth

Which is exactly what this step is all about! Now that you have a better understanding about your limiting seed belief, you can begin to retool the unhelpful seed belief into something that is a better fit for you and your present-day life.

Of course, there are many ways to do this... One way is to rewrite your story, which I cover extensively in my book *Never Too Late: Inspiration and Sage Advice from 7 Later-In-Life Athletes*. Another option is to use active environmental anchors—daily reminders coupled with mental imagery practices that, when used together, create powerful mental and physical conditions for cultivating the seeds of your new, preferred belief. Here are the steps:

**A. Cultivate the preferred belief:** What would you prefer to believe about yourself? Often the preferred belief is the opposite of the unhelpful belief. Not always. It's likely that during the work of the evaluating process, the seed of a preferred, more helpful belief has already started to sprout. What's key here? The new, more helpful belief must feel right to YOU! Write it down using simple, positive language. For example: *I am _____ / I can be _____.* Personal example: *I am fine.*

**B. Collect evidence:** Now it's time to collect evidence to support your new seed belief.

Personal example: *I have the tools and resources I need to take care of this. I will drink more water. I will schedule a massage. I will add in some easy running. I can control many elements here. I will heal. I will be fine.*

## Step 8: More noticing

Back to noticing… Again, get out of the thinking brain and connect with the body brain. Reread your new, more helpful belief statement/s. Stack your answers. How does the body feel now? Again, no right, wrong, or judgement here.

Personal example: *Lighter. Positive. More hopeful.*

## Step 9: Germinate

Now you have a clear understanding (cognition) and sense in your body (nervous system) about your new, preferred belief. It's time, like the dandelion, to let those seeds blow into the wind, germinate, and sprout into new life. There are several ways to do this; the methods below can be very effective.

- *Daily environmental reminders*: Basically, plaster your environment with your preferred seed belief. I love Post-it notes. Write your simple "I am____" preferred belief statement on notes and stick them in strategic places: mirror, car, laptop, by your bed, etc. The point is for your eyes, brain, and nervous system to begin to see, register, and internalize this new—preferred—information multiple times a day.

- *Technology*: Take a snapshot of a sticky note and add your new belief as a screen saver to your phone, laptop, tablet, etc.

Our minds are incredibly powerful. It's no coincidence that many athletes and high performers use mental imagery, or visualization, to enhance their lives. And, thanks to advances in neuroscience, we now have evidence that supports this practice. Researchers Leon Skottnik and David E. J. Linden (2019), in their article published in *Frontiers in Psychiatry*, reviewed the literature covering mental imagery and brain regulation. They confirm that, "repeated positive imagery has been shown to increase the tendency to interpret ambiguous situations as more positive and induce positive mood." Another more current article by Ryan Elder and Aradhna Krishna (2021) also endorses "the central role that mental imagery plays in everyday behavior as well as in human mental function."

I have experienced the benefits of mental imagery, both professionally with people I work with, and personally for healing (psychological and physical), minor surgeries, stress reduction, public speaking, performance enhancement, and even decision making. I would love to delve more deeply into the science behind this fascinating topic, however, I realize that that is beyond the scope of this book.

That said, here are some basic steps you can use to jump-start your mental imagery practice.

## Step 10: Imagery

1. **Space:** You will need a quiet space where you won't be disturbed for ten minutes or   so.

2. **Breath:** Begin to notice your breath, connecting with it wherever/however it shows up in the body. There is no right or wrong here. Just naturally following the breath. In. Out. In. Out. Spend enough time here until you sense your breathing naturally settle down.

3. **Notice:** Begin noticing the body. The sensations: heat/cool, openness/tension, comfort/discomfort, tingling, gurgling, whatever you are actually experiencing in the here and now. **Tip**: Sometimes it helps to mentally label as you notice—tightness, tightness, tightness, warmth, warmth, warmth, tingling, tingling, tingling.

4. **Open:** Be open to whatever arises—as judgement free as possible. Remember, the nervous system communicates through the body. What you are noticing is simply information. Signals. Signposts.

5. **Re-seeding:** Cultivate the new. Using all your work from the steps above: the old limiting belief, your preferred belief, the present-day supporting evidence, and your new "I am" statement. Bring to mind a version of you with your new, preferred belief. A classic

way to do this is to imagine a movie theatre. You are sitting back, relaxing as you watch a version of you embodying your preferred belief. This should include as many of the senses as possible. For instance, hear what you would be saying, see what you would be doing, feel—on a gut level—how your life would be, or is, different. Make your movie as bright and colorful as possible. Turn up the sound. Replay the best parts over and over again. See yourself soaking up all the fresh information surrounding your preferred belief. If it feels good, comfortable, or appropriate, you can add some light, slow, alternate tapping (see the Resources for information about tapping).

6. **Closing:** Spend a few more moments here allowing your nervous system to see, feel, and connect with these new messages, this new information. When you are ready, gently begin to wrap up the movie with gratitude and compassion, slowly coming back to the breath again. Open your eyes. Sit for a few more moments in stillness. What do you notice? Thoughts? Feelings? Images? Body sensations?

Remember, Rome wasn't built in a day, and neither were our limiting beliefs. Like the roots of the dandelion, they are often firmly embedded.

However, they are not fixed; there is a way through...

This work takes patience, grace, and compassion for yourself. Directing this kind of care to your inner self (nervous system) is important. In the beginning, I suggest you repeat this practice/exercise a couple of times a day. In the morning, preferably first thing. In the evening, before or in bed. These are both powerful times—windows when the nervous system is particularly receptive to new information. Also, remember to look at your environmental reminders.

There is a lot of information packed into this chapter. It might be one of those things you read and reread several times. I'd like to emphasize that we are *all* messy humans with messy lives. That's okay. You are okay.

The key take-away here, particularly in our own personal healing and recovery journeys, is to gently nudge our mental/emotional balance from closed, shutdown, and stuck to a more open, broad, fluid view of ourselves and the world—with kindness, curiosity, and compassion. Move away from our all or nothing thinking, limiting beliefs, and knee-jerk reactions toward more balance, present-day truth, and skillful responses that better serve ourselves, our communities, and, frankly, our planet.

We each have been gifted with this incredible human body, brain, and nervous system. We get to live each day on—with—this awe-inspiring planet. We are literally each moment held in the embrace of gravity. We are nurtured and kept alive by the trees, air, water, and what the earth produces. We are an integral part of a vast, limitless universe.

I believe it's deeply human to want to discover, explore, and connect with our external world. The planet. Nature. In the same vein, I encourage a similar curiosity and wonder about our internal worlds; to develop some insight, understanding, and collaboration with what's under the hood or running the show or making us tick. In sum, how can we truly begin to honor our unique, short, precious human lives without embarking on these inner and outer adventures?

———

# WHY NATURE...?

*"In every walk with nature one receives far more than he seeks."*

– John Muir

IT'S NEW YEAR'S EVE morning as I contemplate writing this final chapter. The warmth of primrose and buttermilk shards of light are breaking through the heavy blanket of grey that covers this part of the world in early winter. I sit noticing the movement, the colors, the shapes, the landscape. Even the sounds—almost a hint of spring birdsong somewhere off in the woods.

In this moment I notice I am immersed in a sense of "enoughness." Contentment. I have nowhere to be. Nothing to prove. Nothing to improve. Nothing to optimize. Nothing to compare or compete with. Right now, in this moment, I am, and my life is enough.

Now, outside that moment, I am self-reflecting. I have let the dog out, put away the holiday wrapping and ribbons, wiped the seemingly perpetual crumbs off the kitchen counter, and fired up the laptop. I am aware that the earlier moment of contentment, of course, has passed—yet the feeling, the sense, the realization lingers a little. There is still a taste of enoughness in my body. In my mind. In my nervous system.

Ever had a great massage? Imagine wonderful warm lotion soothing sore, overextended fascia (the tissue that surrounds and holds every organ, blood vessel, bone, nerve fiber, and muscle in place). You get off the table, take a moment to move out of massage brain, so you can pay and drive home. The massage is over. Yet, the effects linger. Compounding. Strengthening. Deepening at a cellular level. That's how that enoughness moment felt. Feels. And that's also why nature…

Nature connects us with a vastness. Our vastness. The awe and wonder of it all. Life. Death. Existence. In nature, if we allow it, time gets lost. Slows. Settles. Becoming more like a rhythm—rising, falling—than a commodity. Ticking. Hurried. Scarce. The natural world tolerates, holds, and accepts. Nature allows our imperfections. Our grief. Our losses. Our traumas. Our messy humanness. Our mistakes.

The concept of holding—and being held—is an important one. Take a moment. Close your eyes and consider being held. Really being held, wrapped up in a warm, soft blanket filled with love. What comes up? Thoughts, feelings, memories, images, longing, warmth, pain? Maybe a lot? Maybe not so much? Either way, it's okay.

It's a fact that baby mammals, in the natural world, will not survive without being tended to. Fed. Warmed. Protected. This need to be nurtured is deeply wired into our DNA. It is a matter of survival. Over time we have seen stories about young children—babies, toddlers—being left or hurt or lost, being found, and cared for by other mammals. Dogs. Gorillas. Bears. Sadly, we also know what happens to baby mammals when they are left alone. Abandoned. Discarded.

To be attended to. To be nurtured. Loved—that's our human word for it. To hold and be held is vital for humans.

Is that the power of nature? Of the natural world? Can nature hold us? Nurture us? Restore our weary souls? Soothe our wounds? Calm our overactive nervous systems? Remind us about the vastness that we are so out of touch with? Connect us with contentment and our enoughness? I say, "Yes!"

At its core, this is what this book is about. The sharing of these courageous stories, experiences, concepts is an invitation to open yourself. To allow yourself—and all your stuff: the good, the bad, and the ugly—to be held. Welcomed. Honored. To be held by the mountains, the plains and prairies, the forests, the streams and oceans, the sky. It's an invitation to step out of those unhelpful stories, the wounds we have all inherited, and the beliefs that limit us. It's about nurturing, holding, opening, seeing moments of space when your enoughness—regardless of the crap you may be swimming in—can shine through. It's about nurturing your body, your mind, your heart. It's about seeing beyond the grief, the loss, the trauma, and the wounds.

Of course, none of this is easy. Yet, paradoxically, it's also not so hard. Think back to childhood. Did time stand still? Endless summer days? The birthday that couldn't arrive fast enough. Other memories? If you have small children around, take a look at them. Notice the wonder. The awe. The excitement. The curiosity. The creativity. The freedom to think, feel, move, express. That's it. Right there. We have that too...

As adults, sadly, much of this has been squeezed out of us by family, school, our performance-driven fear-based culture, and the incessant drip of scarcity messages: not enough time, money, success, love—the list is endless.

In all this, we lose sight; we can't see the forest for the trees. Which means, according to the *Collins Dictionary*, "[we are so] involved in the details of something and so [we] do not notice what is important about the thing as a whole." We have this life, yet are we living it? With it? In it?

Through these pages you have connected with some real people, just like you and me, who courageously shared their inspiring stories. You have heard, first-hand, how they navigated their healing journeys, how they connected with, and moved through, the messiness of it all. The impossible circumstances. The pain. The despair. To discover, or rediscover, the possibilities, hope, even joy life has to offer.

If you have unresolved wounds, pain, or simply feeling a bit lost or disconnected, then I invite you to try connecting with a natural, nurturing space. Consider allowing Mother Nature to hold you, tend to you, soothe you—even for a moment.

Of course, movement matters too, yet it doesn't have to be a 100-mile walk or run or ride. It can be as simple as a few steps around the block, through the local park or green space. Somewhere you can see and be with the natural world. Maybe slowly, over time you too will begin to notice an opening—a moment of enoughness—as you begin to heal and reclaim your life, your creativity, your freedom, your sense of awe in you as a human and the vast, limitless world around you.

———

# RESOURCES

*"Awareness is the first step in healing..."*
— Dean Ornish

I REALIZE THE ROAD to healing—to doing the work—can, at first, seem daunting. Although not exhaustive, consider this chapter a helping hand, if or when you need it. In the interest of accessing information quickly, the resources are categorized by need: anxiety, grief, trauma, addiction, etc. You will find some of the resources highlighted in the interviews, along with other information—websites, books, groups, etc.—that I have, both professionally and personally, found useful. Although focused on the United States, where possible, I have included international resources (note: websites were current at the time of writing).

As I continue to learn, grow, and move through my own grief and trauma, remembering a couple of things has been helpful:

- Taking a tiny step is always better than nothing.
- Getting outside. Remembering to look up and really notice—consider—the vastness of it all.

- Finding a trusted other—for me, a therapist—has been life changing.
- Never give up!

Additionally, today we have a mountain of science-backed evidence to support what we naturally feel or connect with when we are outdoors—particularly in the forest. There are good reasons that being among the pines was, and is, an important part of my healing process. One reason, a no-brainer, is that trees are oxygen producing machines. During those runs and hikes, I was simply getting more oxygen into my body. The second, more recent discovery, is that evergreens (pines, spruce, fir, etc.) produce and release phytoncides into the air. Phytoncides are a natural chemical known to reduce stress hormones, boost white-blood cell count, and support improved immune function. Unbeknown to me, between the movement, the oxygen, and the phytoncides, I was doing more for my health than I realized. Thank you, Mother Nature!

Lastly, because I am a people helper, and, over the years, I have had my share of personal therapy experiences, I know accessing care can be challenging and feel overwhelming—something that's not helpful when you're not at your best. I compiled a *free* downloadable resource to help support you through the process of seeking a helping relationship. *How to Find a Therapist* contains information about the plethora of "therapy" options available today: counseling, coaching, inpatient, outpatient, psychiatry, etc.; what to expect on your first appointment; therapeutic fit and why it's important; plus other tips. Please feel free to use and share as needed.

**Addiction**

*Alcoholics Anonymous* (AA) is an international fellowship of alcoholics dedicated to sobriety and recovery through its spiritually-inclined "Twelve Steps" program. Membership and participation are free. A Google search can connect you with an online or in-person meeting every day, 24/7. You can show up and simply listen. In my opinion, the power of AA is honesty, acceptance, and community.

*SMART Recovery* is an international non-profit organization that provides assistance to individuals seeking abstinence from addiction. SMART stands for Self-Management and Recovery Training. A Google search can connect you with information, meetings, along with other tools and strategies.

*The Substance Abuse and Mental Health Services Administration* (SAMHSA) is a branch of the US Department of Health and Human Services. Here you can find resources about getting help, suicide prevention, substance abuse, and behavioral health.

There is also a National Helpline at (800) 662-HELP (4357).

## Alternative Healing Approaches

*Sacred Medicine: A Doctor's Quest to Unravel the Mysteries of Healing* by Lissa Rankin, MD. This resource-rich guide widens the lens of traditional Western medicine's view of health and healing to include exploration into alternative healing practices from around the world.

*No Bad Parts: Healing Trauma and Restoring Wholeness with the Internal Family Systems Model* by Richard Schwartz, PhD. Dr. Schwartz is the founder of the Internal Family Systems (IFS) model of psychotherapy. This book helps readers recognize and shift their often harsh internal "voices" to new ways of understanding and relating to their inner selves with curiosity and compassion.

## Anxiety/depression

*The American Counseling Association* (ACA) is a non-profit organization that strives to support professional counselors, and grow and strengthen the field of counseling, mental health, and addictions. Here you can access a Therapy Directory of well qualified Licensed Mental Health Professionals.

Website: https://www.counseling.org/aca-community/learn-about-counseling/what-is-counseling/find-a-counselor

*The American Psychiatric Association* (APA) is the main professional organization of psychiatrists and trainee psychiatrists in the United States. Here you can access a comprehensive list of resources and information for patients and families.

Website: https://www.psychiatry.org/patients-families

*The Anxiety and Depression Association of America* (ADAA) is a US nonprofit organization dedicated to increasing awareness and improving the diagnosis, treatment, and cure of anxiety and depressive disorders in children and adults. Their website includes education, information, and other helpful links.

Website: https://adaa.org/

**Grief/Loss/Suicide**

*The American Foundation for Suicide Prevention* (AFSP) is a voluntary health organization based in New York City. The organization's stated mission is to "save lives and bring hope to those affected by suicide." Here you can find information, support, and resources both nationally (US) and internationally.

Website: https://afsp.org/

*The Centre for Addiction and Mental Health* (CAMH) is a psychiatric teaching hospital located in Toronto, Canada. Their website offers a wide array of resources and information with a focus on grief and a variety of loss (home, job, school, etc.).

Website: https://www.camh.ca/

*The Centers for Disease Control and Prevention* (CDC) is the national public health agency of the United States. Here you can access information, education, and resources on many topics including grief and loss.

Website:
https://www.cdc.gov/mentalhealth/index.htm


**How to Find a Therapist**

*BetterHelp*—One of the struggles with the COVID pandemic has been access to care. Organizations like BetterHelp, an online portal that provides direct-to-consumer access to mental health services, have been beneficial. BetterHelp offers counseling and therapy services through web-based interaction as well as phone and text communication.

Website: https://www.betterhelp.com/

*How to Find a Therapist* by Kate Champion is a no-cost downloadable resource which can be found at the author's website.

Website:
https://katechampionauthor.com/resources/

*Psychology Today*—From behavioral research to practical guidance on relationships, mental health, addictions, to making an appointment, this international platform allows you to search, read profiles, and connect with helping professionals worldwide.

Website: https://www.psychologytoday.com/intl

## Mindfulness/Meditation

*Eckhart Tolle: Essential Teachings with Oprah Winfrey*—A helpful podcast, particularly Episodes 1 through 10 where the hosts (Tolle and Winfrey) discuss and break down Tolle's book, *A New Earth: Awakening to Your Life's Purpose.*

*Mindful-Based Stress Reduction* (MBSR)—Developed by Jon Kabat-Zin, the link gives access to online mindfulness resources and a MBSR training course which is 100 percent free. The course, open to anyone, was created by a fully certified MBSR instructor, and is based on the program founded by Jon Kabat-Zinn at the University of Massachusetts Medical School.

Website: https://palousemindfulness.com/

*Waking up* an app by Sam Harris. An extensive meditation platform described as "life-changing" by many subscribers. Available for download on Apple and Android.

*The Wise Heart: A Guide to the Universal Teachings of Buddhist Psychology* by Jack Kornfield. In *The Wise Heart* author, psychologist, and Buddhist teacher Jack Kornfield offers an accessible, comprehensive, and illuminating guide to Buddhist psychology. The author believes we all have within us unlimited capacities for extraordinary love, joy, communion with life, and the natural world.

## Movement/Exercise

*Exercised: Why Something We Never Evolved to Do is Healthy and Rewarding* by Daniel Lieberman. If exercise is healthy, why do many people dislike or avoid it? A book of engaging stories and explanations that will revolutionize the way you think about exercising—not to mention sitting, sleeping, sprinting, weightlifting, playing, fighting, walking, jogging, and even dancing.

*Dopamine Nation: Finding Balance in the Age of Indulgence* by Anna Lembke, MD. This book is about pleasure. It's also about pain. Most important, it's about how to find the delicate balance between the two, and why now more than ever finding balance is essential.

## Nature

*Braiding Sweetgrass: Indigenous Wisdom, Scientific Knowledge, and the Teachings of Plants* by Robin Wall Kimmerer. A botanist, trained to ask questions about nature through the lens of science, and a member of the Citizen Potawatomi Nation, the author embraces the notion that plants, animals, and trees are our oldest teachers.

*Lifestyle by Nature: One Woman's Break from the Unhealthy Herd to Roam Forever Healthy in Nature's Lifestyle Change Herd* by Betty Holston Smith, Ed.D. This book was written by Dr. Betty, who, as you learned about earlier in this book, has been living according to nature's principles for over 50 years. Dr. Betty, now in her 8th decade, remains injury and disease free, while continuing to run more than 80 miles a week.

*The Hidden Life of Trees: What They Feel, How They Communicate—Discoveries from a Secret World* by Peter Wohlleben. The author shares his deep love of the woods and forest along with groundbreaking discoveries about how trees are like human families: tree parents live together with their children, communicate with them, support them as they grow, share nutrients with those who are sick or struggling, and even warn each other of impending dangers.

*The International Society of Nature and Forest Medicine* (INFOM*)* supports progress and the development of research involving nature and forest medicine, INFOM works to advance nature and medicine as well as contributing to health, welfare, and integrated medical care. INFOM currently maintains ownership of nature and forest medicine scientific data both involving human stress reduction and the accompanying increased activation of human natural killer (NK) cells related to time spent in the natural forest.

Website: https://www.infom.org/aboutus/

*To Speak for the Trees: My Life's Journey from Ancient Celtic Wisdom to a Healing Vision of the Forest* by Diana Beresford-Kroeger. The author gives us deep insights into the hidden life of trees, the healing power of nature, our relationship to forests, and the fundamental importance of forests to our survival. She also shares her Bioplan (to which I have personally committed) which encourages people to join together in replanting the global forest.

*Upstream: Selected Essays* by Mary Oliver (1935-2019) is a beautiful collection of essays from this poet. From the first pages this book oozes love, compassion, and connection while helping to remind us that we are, for a short time, an integral part of something more vast.

## Relationships

*A Healing Space: Befriending Ourselves in Difficult Times* by Matt Licata, Ph.D. Of course, how we relate to ourselves is of the utmost importance. The author invites us to explore our relationship with our inner world—thoughts, beliefs, narratives—with kindness and curiosity.

*The Gottman Institute,* founded by John and Julie Gottman. Their mission is to "reach out to families in order to help create and maintain greater love and health in relationships." Through this website resources, services, and training are available to a broad spectrum of people, families, and professionals.

Website: https://www.gottman.com/

## Stroke/Traumatic Brain Injury

*My Stroke of Insight: A Brain Scientist's Personal Journey* by Jill Bolte Taylor, Ph.D. This powerful memoir narrates the author's journey through a massive stroke (in the left hemisphere of her brain) where she observed her own mind completely deteriorate to the point that she could not walk, talk, read, write, or recall any of her life, all within the space of four brief hours. It offers the reader a unique perspective on the brain and its capacity for healing and recovery.

*National Aphasia Association* (NAA) is a non-profit organization founded in 1987. It is the first national organization dedicated to advocating for persons with aphasia and their families, with resources, support, and information readily accessible at their website.

Website: https://www.aphasia.org/

## Trauma

*The Body Keeps the Score: Brain, Mind, and Body in the Healing of Trauma by* Bessel van der Kolk, M.D. I have recommended this book over and over again as an access point for people as they begin to learn about trauma and recovery. The author walks the reader through science and innovative treatment options such as neurofeedback, mindfulness techniques, play, and yoga.

*Eye Movement Desensitization Reprocessing International Association* (EMDRIA) provides access to an international database of highly-skilled mental health professionals who are trained in Eye

Movement Desensitization Reprocessing (EMDR). EMDR therapy is an extensively researched, effective psychotherapy method proven to help people recover from trauma and other distressing life experiences, including PTSD, anxiety, depression, and panic disorders. (Full disclosure: at the time of writing, I am certified in EMDR and a member of EMDRIA.)

Website: https://www.emdria.org/

*National Center for Post-Traumatic Stress Disorder* provides access to information, support, and education for PTSD and traumatic stress, through the US Department of Veterans Affairs.

Website: https://www.ptsd.va.gov/index.asp

**Violence/Domestic Violence**

*Centers for Disease Control and Prevention* (CDC). Violence is an urgent public health problem, which affects people in all stages of life and can lead to physical, mental, and economic problems. This website offers many resources to help with everything from firearm safety to elder abuse.

Website: https://www.cdc.gov/violenceprevention/index.html

*The National Domestic Violence Hotline.* Call, text, or chat any time to access highly-trained, expert advocates who offer free, confidential, and compassionate support, crisis intervention information, education, and referral services in over 200 languages.

Website: https://www.thehotline.org/

*The United Nations* is an intergovernmental, international organization aiming to maintain peace and security, develop friendly relations among nations, achieve international cooperation, and be a center for human rights and freedom.

Website: https://www.un.org/en/coronavirus/what-is-domestic-abuse

———

# ACKNOWLEDGEMENTS

MY DEEPEST GRATITUDE goes to you, dear reader, and the amazing people who had the courage to share their deeply personal stories in the spirit of supporting and inspiring others. My hope is that through you, and our interconnectedness, this book will find its way into the hands and hearts of those who need a glimmer of hope, support, care, and encouragement—things, at times, we all need as we travel this road called life.

Life takes a team, a village—writing and publishing a book is no different. My sincere thanks go out to my editor Helen Baggott, whose endless patience and professionalism have been invaluable in shaping and polishing the words within these pages. To Doug Heatherly, Ph.D. and the folks at Lighthouse24 design, thank you for your expertise and meticulous eye for detail.

My heartfelt thanks go to my awesome early reader team: Rae Antenucci, Diedre Brainerd, Annie Bush, Elora Canne, Aimee Delorey, Bill Sauer, and Dianne Guidry. Dianne, also an editor, went the extra mile with me during the final review of the manuscript. To each and every one of you "thank you" for your time, your energy, your support, your feedback, and for who you as people. You are the best!

On a professional note, I continue to be humbled and astounded by the courage of the people I have encountered over two decades through my work as a psychotherapist. The determination it takes to start the healing process, to show up, to dig through the muck, and work on self-discovery week after week is profound. To serve in this way has been a privilege and honor. My sincere thanks.

Lastly, I am forever grateful for my inner circle of close friends, which include a handful of wonderful women—trail buddies—who are always up for an adventure. Huge hugs to my family: my two adult children—Benjamin and Miranda—who have and continue to inspire and teach me so much. To my brother Sean who has an uncanny ability to make me laugh. And my husband Mark—thank you for filling my life with light, love, and beautiful music.

———

# FINAL WORDS

AS AN EARTH SIGN (I am a Taurus), I intrinsically have a strong connection with the natural world. That said, writing and researching this book has profoundly deepened that connection and the understanding that we are all—animals, humans, plants, trees—interconnected in ways we cannot imagine. For me, especially in times of struggle, remembering this offers a glimmer of solace. I know I am not alone, and neither are you.

I love these words from Leo Buscaglia (1924–1998):

> *"Too often we underestimate the power of a touch, a smile, a kind word, a listening ear, an honest compliment, or the smallest act of caring; all of which have the potential to turn a life around."*

I invite you to share these stories of hope and healing with loved ones and strangers alike, to get outside and enjoy this amazing planet, and to keep moving, healing, and growing.

The power of community is important; please, if you haven't already, check out the Resources where you can access everything from books to websites to podcasts. Do you need a bit more support getting outdoors—hiking, running, backpacking? Then I encourage you to join our wonderful group of likeminded people at *Back of the Pack Athlete:* https://www.facebook.com/groups/120829418591397

If you like audio, I also have a podcast, *Living Big Mindfully*, where you can hear candid, inspirational conversations with real people about healing, aging, growing, and all the mess and wonder that comes along with life.

Finally, please feel free to connect with me directly at https://katechampionauthor.com; sign up for the *Author Happenings Newsletter* and find other books such as *Never Too Late: Inspiration, Motivation, and Sage Advice from 7 Later-in-Life Athletes*. While you are there remember to download your *FREE* copy of *A Pocket Guide to Hiking, Running & Backpacking—Safety Tips and Strategies: For You—and the Folks Back Home*, check out the podcast, or simply drop me a line—I'd love to hear from you.

Until next time…

———

# READY FOR MORE INSPIRATION...?

*"I devoured this book! Highly recommended—inspiration to achieve your athletic goals at any age."* – Cheryl T.

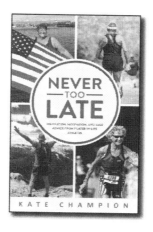

*"I absolutely loved reading stories about older athletes who are still crushing it! I find myself rereading it whenever I need a boost."* – Beth A.

*"If you are hesitant to try something you've always wanted to do, please read this book!"* – Gay S.

Available in paperback and ebook
**katechampionauthor.com**
Download today!

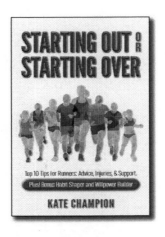

# HERE'S YOUR FREE POCKET GUIDE!

*Whether you are running around town, heading out for your first hike, or trekking in the backcountry—this is the book for you!*

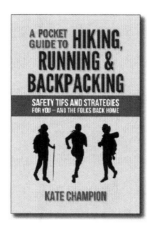

*Efficient, practical, and full of tips— from first aid to trusting your gut!*

Available in paperback and ebook
**katechampionauthor.com**
Download **FREE** today!

Made in the USA
Columbia, SC
21 March 2023

14111615R00154